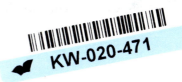

This book is a publication of the International Course in Food
Science and Nutrition (ICFSN). Another publication originating
from this course is:

Selection of technology for food processing in developing
countries, by Domien H. Bruinsma et al. Published by Pudoc, 1983.

Manual for social surveys
on food habits and consumption
in developing countries

Adel P. den Hartog and
Wija A. van Staveren

 Pudoc Wageningen 1983

The authors are lecturers at the Department of Human Nutrition of the
Agricultural University in Wageningen, the Netherlands.

CIP-GEGEVENS

Hartog, Adel, P. den

Manual for social surveys on food habits and consumption in developing
countries / Adel P. den Hartog and Wija A. van Staveren ; (publ. of the
International Course in Food Science and Nutrition (ICFSN)). - Wageningen :
Pudoc. - Ill. Eerder verschenen o.d.t.: Field guide on food habits and food
nutrition. - Wageningen : International Course in Food Science and Nutrition,
1979. - Met lit. opg.
ISBN 90-220-0838-X
SISO 628.44 UDC 641(1-773):303.6
Trefw. : voeding ; ontwikkelingslanden ; enquêtes.

ISBN 90 220 0838 X

© Centre for Agricultural Publishing and Documentation (Pudoc), Wageningen,
1983.

Printed in the Netherlands.

Contents

Preface

This manual on food habits and food consumption is addressed to people with either practical or academic training in nutrition and who are involved in various types of food and nutrition programmes such as nutrition education, supplementary feeding for vulnerable groups, school feeding or applied nutrition programmes. It provides a theoretical background on food habits (Chapters 2-8) and practical information on small surveys on how to collect information on food habits and food consumption.

The material presented is based on the authors' experiences while working with the Food and Agriculture Organization of the United Nations (FAO), Netherlands bilateral aid programmes and with the International Course in Food Science and Nutrition in Wageningen. It is a revised edition of the: 'Field Guide on Food Habits and Food Consumption'.

Many thanks are due to those who have helped in preparing the manual. In particular we would like to thank Ms Wil M. van Steenbergen of the Royal Tropical Institute, Amsterdam.

1 Introduction

This guide provides advice for small-scale surveys on how to collect information on food habits and food consumption and is primarily intended for field staff of food and nutrition programmes in Third World communities such as nutritionists and home-economists. Many of them may feel the need to collect some information on food habits and food consumption during their work in order to throw light on a nutritional problem in their community and to find ways of solving it. Some might not have the necessary experience in conducting social surveys.

The aim of the field guide is to outline how to collect information on food habits and food consumption. Such information may be used:
- For a general reconnaissance of the social context of food and nutrition of a community, its food habits and food consumption. Such a general reconnaissance is needed if one has to deal with a community where hardly any information is available. There is some evidence that even in long-established food and nutrition programmes much basic information is lacking.
- For a more specific problem-oriented approach on food habits and food consumption. Information may be used for anthropometric, clinical or biochemical assessment of the nutritional resources of a population, as indication of who is malnourished and why. The guide may well be used together with the field guide for the assessment of nutritional health prepared by de Wijn (1978). Specific information on food habits and food consumption may be needed during planning, implementation and evaluation of food and nutrition programmes.

The user of the guide should bear in mind that a survey only makes sense if one carefully defines its purpose: the goals of the inquiry, why and what one wants to know. So suggestions and questions, questionnaires and work sheets provided by the Field

Guide should be adapted to the specific aims and needs of the user. One cannot prepare a standard questionnaire on food habits and consumption for every situation.

This publication is intended as a guide and not as a set of rules on food habits and food consumption. It may contain questions not relevant nor applicable to a specific population and nutritional problem. It is not intended as an introduction on how to carry out social surveys and epidemiological studies, which are beyond its scope.

To understand and correct nutrition in a group of people, one must investigate the socio-economic and cultural variables that influence food habits. The nutrition of a group of people is influenced by a wide range of variables such as climate, topography, flora, fauna, population growth, composition of the household, systems of producing crops and livestock, marketing, ownership of land, support, industries and trade, purchasing power, political structure and cultural patterns. The relevance of each variable differs from society to society. Problems of nutrition should not be examined in isolation. During a survey, and in the analysis and interpretation of findings, one must interprete and assess questions of food and nutrition in the light of socio-economic and cultural variables.

2 Introduction to food habits and food consumption patterns

2.1 SOCIAL FUNCTIONS OF FOOD IN SOCIETY

The main function of food in a society is for survival. Social scientists such as Malinowsky (1944) and Richards (1939) pointed out that the human body's need for food has done much to shape society through all the activities concerned with food production, distribution and utilization. Man's interest in food cannot, however, be explained only by an innate biological impulse. De Garine (1971), in a stimulating paper on social and cultural aspects of food habits said that: "Certain nutritionists would have us to believe that nourishment is the ranking pre-occupation of the human species; numerous societies must resort to their utmost ingenuity merely to subsist in a hostile environment, but the importance they attach to nourishment and good eating can vary considerably". Man does not think of his foods in terms of energy and nutrients. Lévi-Strauss suggested that animals just eat food, but that for man society decreed what was food and what was not food and what kind of food should be eaten and on what occasions (Leach, 1970). It is outside the scope of this guide to deal with Lévi-Strauss and his culinary triangle on the opposition between raw, cooked and decayed foods. He considered the art of cooking a major aspect of the civilization of a society.

Besides scientific classification of foodstuffs, people in many societies have traditional ways of classification. In some Philippino communities, people classify their foodstuffs in three different categories: foodstuffs that allay ones hunger such as rice, foodstuffs to satisfy appetite (meat, green leafy vegetables) and taste (salt, peppers).

In many cultures, food may be classed hot or cold by a classification irrelevant to an outsider but deep-seated in the understanding of the community. Ingham (1970) describes a typical three-course rural meal in Mexico beginning with rice (cold), followed by a soup of hot and cold ingredients and ending with dark beans (hot). The contrast of hot and cold foods in present Latin America has its origins in Classical Spanish medicine, and in the indigenous cultures that preceded the Spanish conquest (Molony, 1975). A hot/cold dichotomy is also known in the folk medicine of China, Burma, India and Sri Lanka.

A better knowledge of the social aspects of food and food consumption patterns is useful to understand the nutritional situation of a group of people (Guthe & Mead, 1945). The definition given by Mead (1945) on food habits is clear and practical: "Food habits are the ways in which individuals or groups of persons, in response to social and cultural pressures, choose, consume and make use of available foods."

In nutrition education, one must study the role of food in a particular society. It is therefore useful to distinguish the following interrelated social functions of food in society:
- Gastronomic function
- Means of cultural identity
- Religious and magic function
- Means of communication
- Expressions of economic wealth and status
- Means to exercise influence and power.

2.2   GASTRONOMIC FUNCTION

It is not always fully realized and appreciated but man also eats food for his pleasure. The organoleptic properties of a food can decide whether people accept or reject a food. The pleasure of a food perceived by the human senses is determined by taste, odour, temperature, appearance, structure or texture. The pleasure obtained from food has partly a psychological and cultural basis (Kouwenhoven, 1970). Taste and appreciation of food differs from region to region. People in Europe generally like soft types of food whereas people in tropical Africa like to chew foods, such as meat. In many rice-consuming countries of Asia, there is a taste for a granular structure of the boiled rice. In other parts of the world, glutinous staples are highly appreciated.

The art of cooking and eating should not be overlooked for its positive or negative influence on the nutrition of a society. People can be rather emotional towards their food. Rejecting the food of a community or a country means more than just rejecting a foodstuff.

In the industrial societies, consumers sometimes complain of a tendency for foods, both fresh and processed, to have less taste. The long chain between the urban consumers and the food producers is an enormous challenge to the food industry, which must offer safe foods that retain organoleptic qualities and nutrients during processing, especially in countries with a young food industry and an interest in processing traditional foods and dishes for the modern consumer, and in competing with imported foods.

2.3 MEANS OF CULTURAL IDENTITY

Food may establish the cultural identity of a group of people or even a whole nation. For example in the traditional Senegalese society, each group can identify itself and looks at the others through a mesh of taboos and obligations, including food (de Garine, 1962). Among traditional farmers in Mexico, maize is identified with life and attitudes towards it are often religious. Outsiders may identify a community by its foods. The Eskimo people call themselves Inuit, which means people. The name Eskimo, meaning eaters of raw meat, was given to them by their neighbours the Algonquin Indians, referring to their particular food habits.

Food avoidances or taboos in a society serve to show differences between various groups and as a means of cultural identity. In Muslim countries with Christian communities, eating of pork distinguishes the two different groups quite clearly. The same applied until recently in Europe where the eating of fish or meat on a Friday indicated whether people were Roman Catholics or not (Section 6.2)

Industrial society may stimulate new emotional feelings towards food (e.g. Dwyer et al., 1974). The number of "Health Food" shops, selling "natural" products such as foods grown without artificial fertilizers or insecticides, or foods containing no preservatives or artificial colouring, is increasing. Food cults such as those of Hay, Bircher-Benner and Hauser have many follow-ers. It seems that some sections of youth are more to 'macro-biotic' and other special forms of diets (Frankle & Heussenstamm, 1974). Often these diets are rigidly vegetarian and pose prob-lems for nutritional health. They should not, however, be con-fused with the diets of traditional vegetarian communities. There are several reasons why sections of industrial society have accepted these new cults. They may be a protest against the establishment and its environmental problems. They may distin-guish the group from the rest of society and give a feeling of identity.

2.4 RELIGIOUS OR MAGIC FUNCTION

There is much religious or magic symbolism associated with food and these should be analysed within the context of society. The role of food in religion should be taken into account in nutrition education (Sakr, 1971). In many communities, the atti-tude of man towards his staple food has a sacred character, and dietary regulations about food are used in God's service.

Of a quite different nature is the use of food among some groups in magic rituals. In folk medicine, food is considered to have special properties. For example, the consumption of a cer-tain food during pregnancy may be considered harmful for the mother or child.

2.5 FOOD AS MEANS OF COMMUNICATION

Foods offered to a visitor or a guest may put people at ease and facilitate communication. Hospitality is in many countries a heavy burden on the household budget.

The exchange of gifts of food between individuals or groups on social occasions has an important function. Most such meals on social occasions have a strongly competitive element. One example is that of the Kwakiutl Indians on the west coast of North America, who held competitive festivals, the potlatches, where food played an important role. A competitive element prevails too at many dinner parties, weddings and other festivities in Western culture, although this may not be admitted.

In industrial communities where man and wife both work outside the home during the day and the children go to school, the evening meal is often the only occasion where the family is together. So food allows people to communicate.

2.6   FOOD AS AN EXPRESSION OF ECONOMIC STATUS

Food is a sign of wealth or status. All cultures have prestige foods, mainly reserved for special occasions. The eating of white bread was long the privilege of the rich in Europe; the poorer classes ate brown bread.

The increasing contact among countries has often caused Western (e.g. refined or processed) food to be considered as a sign of prestige in less industrial countries. Painter (1972) describes the gradual reduction in fibre in the diet with increased processing of foodstuffs and its implications for the health of industrial societies.

2.7   MEANS TO EXERCISE INFLUENCE AND POWER

Food can be used to exercise influence. Those persons or groups in control of the food supply can also control society. History shows many examples of this. From the beginning of urban life in ancient times, towns have tried to subdue the countryside in order to ensure a steady supply of food. Urban authorities could thus gain political influence over the towns folk, and often also over neighbouring farming communities. In the modern world, food aid to poor countries may be abused as a means of ensuring political influence.

Likewise in the household, food can be used to gain influence by the person responsible for the family store.

3 Food habits and ecology

Food habits are influenced by many environmental variables (Figure 1).

Choice and use of available food have an ecological component. Regional studies under the Indicative Plan for Agricultural Development of FAO (1970) showed a close relation between the diet of a community and the ecological zone where it was situated (see also Annegers, 1973). Domestication of plants in response

Social:
Land tenure
Food production system
Marketing
Purchasing power
Patterns of culture

Physical:
Urban/rural dwellings
Roads
Utensils

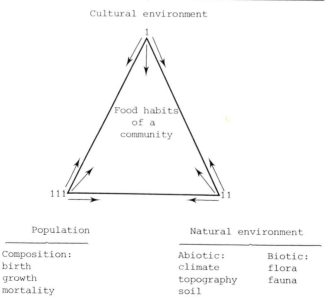

Cultural environment

Food habits
of a
community

Population

Composition:
birth
growth
mortality

Natural environment

Abiotic: Biotic:
climate   flora
topography   fauna
soil

Figure 1. Main variables in food habits of a community.

to natural ecosystems has led to two main cropping systems: seed culture primarily dependent upon crop plants reproduced by seed, and root-and-tuber culture, dependent mainly on vegetative reproduction (Harris, 1969). Seed agriculture is the indigenous mode of agriculture in the drier tropics and subtropics of the Old and New World. Root-and-tuber agriculture is most highly developed as an indigenous agriculture in the humid tropical lowlands of America, South East Asia and Africa. In the highlands of the Andes with a cool temperate climate, root and tuber agriculture is based on potatoes and some minor root crops. Domestication of plants and animals initiated major changes in human ecology, leading to larger settled communities and ultimately to the amenities of urban life.

Plant domestication can also lead to dependence on a single staple, such as rice, maize, cassava or plantain. If this staple is poor in certain nutrients, nutritional deficiencies may result. In the forest zones of tropical Africa with root-and-tuber culture, the diet is characterized by a deficiency of proteins and riboflavin. In the savanna zones of West Africa, deficiencies of riboflavin, and vitamins A and C are common during the long dry season when vegetables are scarce and animal production is limited by scarcity of pasture and other animal fodder. The amount of these nutrients in the staples millet and sorghum, is not sufficient to compensate for these periodic shortages of other foods.

According to Oomen (1971), man can be considered as part of an ecosystem in a dynamic equilibrium that has not been disturbed, even in large population groups. As an example, he shows that the traditional New Guinean diets of the root-and-tuber growers rarely lead to malnutrition. Although communities situated in the same ecological zone usually have a similar dietary pattern, this does not mean that all their food habits are the same. Differences may be found between various communities of the same ecological zones, e.g. in food distribution, food avoidance, infant feeding. The age-old balance of the community with its environment is now being disturbed by external factors.

Geertz (1963) described two types of human ecosystem in Indonesia: Swidden ecosystem (shifting cultivation), and Sawah or

wet-rice ecosystem. The two ecosystems were broken up by external interference. Three main forces causing deterioration in a
balanced ecosystem and in the food habits of a community were
population growth, orientation away from subsistence cropping
towards cash cropping and urbanization.

4 Orientation from subsistence farming to cash-crob farming

4.1 CASH CROPS AND FOOD CROPS

Despite the fact that pure subsistence farming can only be found in remote areas, the foods consumed in many rural coomunities are mainly derived from the consumer's own farm (FAO, 1977a). A vast majority of the Asian population still lives on foods they produce themselves. In Africa south of the Sahara, FAO (1970) estimated that 64% of the food consumed was derived from subsistence farming.

Farming in most developing countries is characterized by production of food crops for household use and crops for sale. Cash cropping can nowadays even be found in remote areas and money has become a necessity of rural life. This cash among country people is needed for several purposes:
- purchase of essential goods such as clothing, soap, matches, salt, sugar, tea, coffee and kerosine;
- to meet social obligations such as dowry, wedding or funeral;
- for provisions such as a school or health centre, even when these provisions are meant to be free of charge;
- to pay taxes to local or central government.

With economic development of rural areas, agriculture becomes directed towards cash crops and marketing. From many points of view, this process is necessary as it gives the country the needed resources for economic development and allows the farmer to raise the standard of living for himself and his family. In many countries, only a small part of the income derived from the rural areas by the government is used for rural development (e.g. Lipton, 1977). This process may have harmful side-effects for nutrition: replacement of labour-intensive food crops by food crops requiring less labour, but nutritionally inferior; replacement of food crops by non-food cash crops.

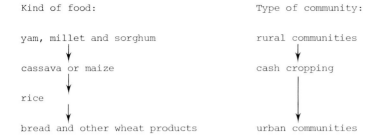

Kind of food:	Type of community:
yam, millet and sorghum ↓	rural communities ↓
cassava or maize ↓	cash cropping
rice ↓	
bread and other wheat products	urban communities

Figure 2. Trends with food stuffs in tropical Africa.

Such side-effects worsen the already weak socio-economic position of small farmers and of agricultural labourers employed on larger farms and plantations. The food supply of rural households becomes dependent on low and irregular wages or returns.

A cash crop may be a food or non-food crop. In many areas food crops needing a lot of work are abandoned for less time-consuming foods such as cassava or maize with a high energy yield. In Africa south of the Sahara there is a tendency to replace yam, millet and sorghum by cassava, maize or rice (Figure 2). Other regions of the world show similar trends. In Mexico and Central America, there is a tendency to replace maize by bread and rice. Everywhere in the world where people have the opportunity, there seems to be a tendency to replace traditional unrefined dark cereal flours by refined white wheat flour or polished white rice, for reasons of taste, convenience and prestige - to the detriment of nutrition.

The cash income of the family is often not used to compensate the lost nutritive value by purchase of additional foods. Investigations in a settlement with irrigated farming in Kenya revealed that the improvement in living standards did not coincide with an improvement in the nutritional status (Kraut & Cremer, 1969). Apparently, other needs such as better clothing, a radio or a bicycle had to be satisfied first.

4.2 WOMEN AND FOOD PRODUCTION

Commercialization of agricultural production has often been detrimental to the position of women. In most rural communities women work with crops or livestock, as well as in the household. Tropical Africa is a good example of what may happen with commercialization, because farmers there are pre-dominantly women (FAO, 1979) (Table 1). Hill (1978) described the situation in West Africa as a symbiotic relationship between husband and wives as cultivators. The husband assists the wife in the heavy agricultural tasks of the farm, such as clearing the fields; the wife assists the husband with weeding. The wife's obligations are to process and cook for the household and to carry firewood and water, perhaps with help from her children. Apart from these tasks, she may usually occupy her time as she wishes, for instance marketing food or other commodities without any obligation to hand over the proceeds to her husband. Cash crops weaken the socio-economic status of women. Agricultural extension is directed to cash crops and to men. The weakened role of women aggravates dietary deficiency in rural households.

4.3 SCARCITY OF FUEL FOR COOKING

Apart from difficulties related to marginal food supplies, low income and rising food prices, poorer households have to

Table 1. *Fraction of labour provided by women in various activities associated with food production and supply in rural tropical Africa. After FAO 1974a.*

food production	0.70*
food storage in the home	0.50
food processing	1.00
animal husbandry	0.50
marketing	0.60
brewing of beer	0.90
water supply	0.90
fuel collection	0.80

* Percentage of total labour associated with a particular task attributed to women and expressed as a fraction of 1.

cope with diminishing sources of fuel (FAO, 1981). In developing countries, most fuel is used for cooking. Only in mountains and high plateaux may fuel be used for heating. The main fuel is usually firewood. In deforested areas where livestock are kept dung may be used. Crop residues may be used too. In many societies, it is the task of women and children to collect firewood. According to Eckholm (1976), about 90% of the people in developing countries depends on firewood as their chief source for cooking. Population growth is outpacing the growth of new trees to the nutritional detriment of poorer households in the long term.

Scarcity of fuel may have the following effects.
- The search for firewood, once a task with little difficulty, may become a real burden for women.
- The costs of firewood will increase and therefore add to the total expenditure for food. In urban areas of the Sahel sucn as Ougadougou (Upper Volta), fuel for cooking may cost up 20-30% of an average wage (Eckholm, 1976).
- The intense search for firewood will bring about further deforestation and erosion, and endanger food production.
- The use of cow-dung as a fuel to replace firewood as in the Indian subcontinent, has other long-term consequences for food production and nutrition. Cow-dung is not returned to the soil to provide the organic structure necessary for food production.

Alternative sources of fuel are not easy to find for the poorer households. Kerosine and other fuels are increasingly expensive for households used to collect firewood 'for no cost'. Biogas derived from cow-dung and solar heaters are possible only for better-off households. Some countries try to solve some of these problems by planting fast-growing trees for fuel around urban settlements. Many households still cook on three stones over an open fire. A charcoal pot on the ground or floor. This is a wasteful method, since cooking over an open fire has an energy efficiency of 0,1 (Pimentel & Pimentel, 1979). Stoves made of local materials such as clay or earth are less wasteful of energy.

14

5 Influence of towns on food habits and urbanization

Migration from rural to urban areas is a widespread phenomenon. Before the Industrial Revolution, urbanization was primarily a tendency of the countryfolk to gravitate towards large towns with good administrative and commercial facilities while retaining their farming activities. In modern cities, the agricultural element is negligible.

Many townsfolk are newcomers. As Southall & Gutkind (1957) said of Kampala, they are "townsmen in the making". Urban growth is not only caused by migration, but also by the natural growth of many cities in developing countries (Arriaga, 1968). The migrant coming to the town is faced with many problems: the change from a rural to an urban environment and way of life, finding employment and housing, and the social experience of being separated from his family if the family remains in the village. The new urban environment affects food habits and dietary pattern (Freedman, 1973). In contrast to the countryside, all foods have to be bought. The supply of local traditional commodities is often inadequate and there is not always sufficient time for lengthy food preparation. In the town, the family loses several important economic functions, such as production and preservation of foods, weaving and making clothes. All these factors make townsfolk receptive to new foods that are quick and easy to prepare (bread, sugar, rice) and attractively packed. Most will be preserved foods.

Another aspect of accepting new foods is the growing tendency in urban areas to replace breast-feeding with artificial feeding soon after birth (Section 6.3).

According to de Garine (1969), urban food habits depend first on traditional food habits at home and second on new influences, for instance from eating in workers' canteens.

In Accra, Ghana, new foods were used by migrants to towns but were adapted to their traditional culinary techniques (den Hartog, 1973a).

Despite insufficient employment, overcrowding, inadequate cooking facilities and expensive housing, many comparisons with countryfolk show that townsfolk have
- more varied food, including fruit and vegetables;
- more meat;
- less seasonal influence on diet.
(Bornstein, 1972a; de Garine, 1969; Dema & den Hartog, 1969; Jones, 1963; Santos, 1967). However this general impression is subjective, as the situation may differ from country to country, and between socio-economic groups in one town.

Especially in larger cities, there are often large marginal groups of underemployed or unemployed people with very low and irregular incomes. These groups live in shanty towns that sprung up at the edges of the cities in poor countries. The nutritional problems of the urban poor are different from those of traditional countryfolk.

Surveys in India, Sri Lanka and Brazil show that the urban poor have a lower energy intake than the rural poor (FAO, 1977a). See also Table 2.

Traditional farmers have certain advantages over the citizens of a cash-crop society. Within their limited physical resources, traditional farmers have achieved a social and ecological equilibrium. They can foresee seasonal shortages, hazards of climate and other environmental difficulties, and they have built up traditions as a defence against these. In the urban society, the flow of resources is outside the control of the majority. Unforeseen problems arise and cannot be overcome by experience. For example, developing countries have experienced inflation in prices of foodstuffs, which hits townsfolk much harder than countryfolk, who depends partly on his own production. This may be illustrated by what a Sisala migrant in Accra, Ghana, said (Grindal, 1973) "When I was living with my father, my food was free, my room was free. At home I worked hard on the farm but I never had to worry. Here in Mamobi (Accra) everything

*Table 2. Intake of crude energy by income group in Sri Lanka, 1969/70
(data from FAO, 1977a, Table II.1.4).*

Income (rupees)	Place		Number of households surveyed	Energy rate (MJ/d)
≤ 200	Colombo:	urban	353	10.25
		rural	185	11.92
	other :	urban	471	10.88
		rural	1368	11.09
200 - 399	Colombo:	urban	745	11.92
		rural	264	11.51
	other :	urban	643	11.09
		rural	1076	11.72
400 - 599	urban		682	11.51
	rural		416	12.13
≥600	urban		841	12.34
	rural		196	12.34

costs money. If you cannot find work, you will starve and nobody
cares". In a village community there is usually a system of mu-
tual aid to help members in distress and prevent individuals
from starving. For instance in Yemeni villages, there is a tradi-
tion for families who have milk animals to distribute skim milk
free to poor neighbours who have no animals (Bornstein, 1974).
With the weakening of social ties in urban areas, such protec-
tion against misfortune is weaker, and the individual is more
vulnerable socially and nutritionally.

Closely related to this drastic social change, one may observe an increase in the consumption of alcoholic beverages and
increase in the incidence of alcoholism in many areas. The background of this phenomenon can be explained in the despair to be
found in many towns with unemployment, economic failure and insufficient care and aid by the authorities. In some rural areas,
consumption of alcohol is also increasing. As Obayemi (1976) ob-
serves for rural Nigeria, social changes have created extra op-
portunities for the purchase of alcoholic beverages. To supple-
ment the local products, European types of liquor, either imported or produced locally, are becoming increasingly common

with the idea that it adds to the sophistication of parties and
ceremonies.

5.2   URBAN INFLUENCE ON FOOD HABITS IN RURAL AREAS

The definitions of what constitutes an urban area are many.
In our context, let us take "urban" to mean an area with a
sizeable population (e.g. the lower limit in Ghana is set at
5000 inhabitants), few producing food and most depending on the
market for their food supply.

Urbanization is a two-way process, not only the migration of
people from the rural areas to the cities, but also on outward
spread of urban influence into the rural areas (Anderson, 1964;
Gutkind, 1974). From early times, cities have endeavoured to get
the rural areas under their political and economic control to
ensure the cities food supply. Political power in most countries
is still situated in the cities. Compared with their urban coun-
terpart, the rural population often has less political influence.
One may distinguish two main aspects of urban influence on the
rural areas: "physical" urbanization and "mental" urbanization.
"Physical" urbanization does not only mean the incorporation of
the villages into conurbations but also bringing roads and better
housing. "Mental" urbanization or urbanism introduces rural areas
to the urban way of life and therefore influences the food habits
of rural people.

Urban influence on the food and nutrition of the population
of rural areas may have the following effects (Sections 5.2.1-3).

5.2.1 Migration and rural nutrition

Rural-urban migration presents the danger that the young
able-bodied men leave, reducing the farm labour force and leaving
behind women, children and the elderly. This may endanger the
food economy unless agriculture is modernized to overcome the
loss of labour. This is particularly so in less densely populated
areas as in parts of Malaysia, where the absence of young people
hinders rice production. Though it is often stated that traditional agriculture has a surplus of labour, this is not true

18

with peak demand at certain periods of the year, e.g. during harvest.

With the increased workload borne by rural women when the men are absent, care and feeding of children and cohesion and stability of family life suffer, even though the men show their sense of responsibility by sending large amounts of money to their households back home.

These phenomena have been observed in several parts of the world. A detailed account is given by Adepoju (1974) for urban migrants and their home communities in south-west Nigeria. More than half the migrants send money home from time to time, as well as taking gifts home during visits. A large proportion of the remittances goes in buying food (Table 3). Although most of the food consumed in the rural areas was produced on the farms, farm yields had decreased with the drain of the energetic young people from the farm and the use of traditional techniques by ageing farmers who cultivate marginally fertile land.

Hansen (1970) described how absence from the farm of men

Table 3. Use of remittances sent by urban migrants in the towns of Ife and Oshogbo, Western State of Nigeria, to their relatives in rural areas (Adepoju, 1974).

	Ife		Oshogbo	
	Number	Proportion (%)	Number	Proportion (%)
Number of respondents	369	100	235	100
Maintenance of family				
food	185	50.1	135	57.5
other needs	144	39.1	83	35.3
Education of children	51	13.8	28	11.9
To trade, pay labourers, build a house, repair family house	33	8.9	26	11.1
Others: to meet specific projects	20	5.4	14	5.9

working in an oil refinery harmed the food situation of a Bahrein village. The result for the village as a whole was summarized as follows: less substantial food; smaller harvest of dates and lucerne; very few cows, if any, and so lack of milk for infants. Although the wages were high, they were not well spent from the nutritional point of view.

Hill (1978) mentioned that the absence from the rural community in southern Ghana of the younger men and many of the younger women reduced the efficiency of farming. Because of migration, most farmers were middle-aged or elderly and supply of day-labourers was inadequate. Husband and wife had separate farming tasks. For instance men always cleared the forests and prepared the field, whereas women always weeded and marketed food. Spouseless men and women found it difficult to get someone to do the agricultural work considered appropriate to the opposite sex.

5.2.2 Urban markets and food production

Urbanization directs any food production to the urban market. This will not only result in an increasing demand for staple foods but also for foods such as fruit, vegetables and meat as the income of the townsfolk generally rises faster than of countrymen. Though the farmer's standard of living may rise, there may be harmful side-effects for nutrition. Food crops for marketing in the town may be grown at the expense of food crops for the farmer's own family. Just after harvest, too much of a food crop may be sold at a low price, at the expense of the stocks for home consumption. When food stocks diminish later in the year, food has to be bought back at a higher price.

5.2.3 Spread of urban food habits into the rural areas

The urban influence will cause some of the rural population to adopt elements of the urban food habits.

Good and new ideas adopted in towns spread to the rural areas and influence rural food habits. From the town, commercial activities, radio programmes and newspapers penetrate rural areas. Villagers go to town to sell their commodities and bring back the goods they need, including foods. Many townsfolk have not severed their ties with their home villages, which they visit from time to time (McGee, 1975). Some workers go back to the village for some time and later return to the town. In Bombay, 20-30% of new arrivals go back after some time to their home villages. Some receive food from rural households. Some people consider themselves as only temporarily urban dwellers and later return to their villages. All this indicates close contact between the urban and the rural world. Foods such as soft drinks, tins of milk, fish or meat and sugar, bread and biscuits spread from the towns to rural areas of many tropical countries. Although these foods play a marginal role in the total diet, they are much appreciated for their taste and convenience.

Not all urban influence by far is good. In many villages, the plastic feeding bottle, powdered milk and condensed milk in tins are familiar products, adopted under urban influence and causing serious health problems.

5.3 FOOD HABITS OF SOCIO-ECONOMIC CLASSES

5.3.1 The main urban classes

In towns, one may distinguish three socio-economic classes, which can be subdivided into narrower groups. Each class has characteristic food habits and nutrition (Figure 3). Although middle and high classes are small, their food habits have strong economic consequences, especially their demand for imported foods. In many countries, food imports are a heavy drain on foreign exchange that could otherwise be used for investment.

As yet there is little information on diets of unestablished newcomers to towns, living in shanty towns, spontaneous settlements or bidonvilles. In a Caracas shanty town, fresh meat, green vegetables and milk were unknown. Food resembled that of the countryside, but people no longer ate chicken and fresh fruit as they used to do (Brisseau, 1963). Shanty towns are widely regarded as "sinks of social disorganization", but studies in Peru, for example, showed that the opposite was true in the squatter settlements or "barriadas" (Mangin, 1967). The

FOOD HABITS

High:	High intake of energy, protein, fat
traditional aristocracy; high-ranking	and sugar. Some have unbalanced
civil servants; modern managers	diet through overeating.
	Large intake of imported and conve-
	nience foods
Middle:	Elements of high and low groups.
professional; lower civil servants	Strong tendency to emulate the high
	group.
Low:	Lower intake of energy, protein,
labourers; proletariat; in some cities	fat and sugar.
40-80% of the population	Unbalanced diet through poverty.
	Low intake of imported foods.

Figure 3. Food habits among urban socio-economic classes in developing countries.

people fared better than in city slums: though poor, they did not live a life of squalor and hopelessness (Lloyd, 1979; Gugler et al. 1981).

In Africa, migrants often organized themselves on an ethnic basis, so helping many newcomers to adapt themselves to the new urban situation. Jocano (1975) points out for Metro Manila that people in shanty towns are far from what they are often said to be. Many of them improved themselves despite poverty, environment, "sub-cultural socialization" and other social handicaps. Given the conditions they are in and their meagre skills, it is amazing, how they survive the pressures of urban life. Despite many problems to be found in shanty towns, there are also positive aspects such as the will to survive and to improve life which should be taken into account in planning and implementing nutritional aid (UNICEF, 1982).

In the shanty towns, there are positive elements for workers in nutrition education, while in old urban areas in decay, the

social situation is much more difficult. In some Asian cities,
shanty town dwellers have taken their own initiative in order to
improve their living conditions. Sometimes these shanty town
dwellers managed to force the urban policy-makers to join their
efforts (e.g. UNICEF, 1977).

5.3.2   Rural classes

Many of the differences in food habits between classes in
urban areas apply also to rural areas with distinct social
classes. This does not generally apply to traditional rural
tropical Africa, although differences may be found in regions
with a highly developed cash economy, such as the cocoa-growing
areas in West Africa. Most of rural Latin America and Asia are
quite different. After the land reform of 1952 in Bolivia, the
improvement in living conditions, particularly the nutrition of
peasants, was so marked that the average size of army recruits
increased markedly (Huizer, 1973). More food crops would so become available for household use and peasants simply ate a good
deal better, which was also one of the temporary decrease in
marketed agricultural produce in the first post reform years.
Agrarian reform does not, however, automatically improve the
food and nutrition of the farmer.

A study by Basta (1977) suggested that differences in health
and nutrition between the various urban classes were greater
than between town and country.

5.3.3   Income

Income is a major factor in food habits and nutrition. With
a significant increase of income, more expensive foods are purchased and eaten. Generally, we see a change from starchy staple
foods to more meat, fats, sugars, fruit and vegetables. People
may change from cheaper staple (e.g. cassava) to more expensive
staples such as rice and wheat. With rising income too, the proportion of income spent on food diminishes. This is known as
Engel's law; after the 19th Century statistician Ernst Engel who
observed this phenomenon in Germany. Better-off households spend

no more than 30% of their income on food whereas lower income groups spend more than 70%. Of course, the absolute expenditure on food is much greater among the well-to-do.

Because of this, it is often assumed that people in developing countries will vary their diet more as income rises. This might happen in the long run. However studies carried out in Sri Lanka indicate a quite modest effect of income in changing food habits. Poleman et al. (1973) concluded that long-term improvements in the nutritional status will depend on a faster rate of economic growth and on the speedy provision of more and better jobs for its expanding workforce.

Despite great efforts on development by various governments, income improvement among the lower strata of society has so far been limited.

To understanding the food and nutrition of low-income groups, one must realize that being underprivileged is expensive. Low income forces people to buy small amounts, which are more expensive than larger amounts. Spontaneous settlements or shanty towns are generally situated far from central markets where cheaper foods and other commodities can be bought. Because of the public transport involved, these markets are less accessible to low-income consumers. Fuel for cooking is a relative high burden for low-income households. In some Latin American and Indian cities, traditional tortillas or chapattis are replaced by white bread, not to be modern but because of lack of money to buy fuel (Nelson et al., 1978).

5.3.4 Household size

Household size influences food habits and nutrition, particularly among poor households depending on cash income for the purchase of food. With increase in size of the household, consumption of animal foods decreases and staple foods are replaced by cheaper ones or decrease as well. Intake of energy and protein may decrease (Table 4).

24

Table 4. Household size and rate of intake of energy and protein per person in eight regions of the Philippines. Data from Quioguo et al. (1969).

Number in household	Energy intake		Intake of protein (g/d)
	(MJ)	(kcal)	
1- 3	9.1	2180	66
4- 6	7.3	1750	51
7- 9	6.8	1620	45
10-12	6.7	1600	44
Over 12	6.3	1500	43

6 Food distribution in the household and infant feeding

6.1 FOOD DISTRIBUTION

Food available in a country, whether locally produced or imported, is not evenly distributed between people. Uneven distribution of food is found between different regions of a country,
rural and urban areas, between different socio-economic groups,
and also between members of the household.

Supply and distribution of food in a rural household may be
summarized as in Figure 4, which is based on Lewin's Channel
Theory. In a survey, one must find out which members of the
household control the various channels: the husband, wife or domestic staff. In some societies, the housewife is responsible
for buying and the husband for supply from the farm. The women
may control supply from the farm for vegetables and the men for
staple foods, as in various parts of tropical Africa. In Yemen

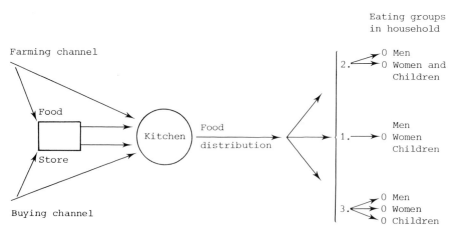

Figure 4. Supply and distribution of food in a rural household. After den
Hartog (1973).

26

and other traditional Muslim societies, it is usually the men who buy food and who control the household budget (Bornstein, 1972).

Members of a household will not always eat together around the same "table" as in most Western societies. In other parts of the world, members of the household may eat in separate groups and not all at the same time. In Indonesia, men eat first, and women and children later; in parts of Africa, there are sometimes three eating groups: the men, the women and very young children, and the other children under the guidance of an older sister.

One must find out which group receives the food first, and who is responsible for apportioning the food not only as a whole but also in the various eating groups.

Apportionment of food has both a physiological and socio-cultural basis. Important socio-cultural factors influencing it are as follows:
- social status in the household; who has the first choice of the food; sequence in which meals are served
- prevailing concept toward food
- social function of food, especially food as an expression of prestige, and the obligations of hospitality.

In societies with male dominance, it is common that meat is to a certain extent regarded as belonging to men and it is also a means for men to reinforce his prestige (den Hartog, 1973 b).

In many cultures, food sharing and food gifts have a strong social and religious significance. In Islam, eating is considered to be a matter of worship of God, like praying, fasting and other religious practices, It is said that the amount of food for one person is always enough for two, and the amount for two is enough for four; it is unthinkable that a person should eat his food alone without sharing it with other people present.

Food gifts are a way of showing one's friendship and appreciation of a person or compassion for the poor. The sharing of meat during the Islamic Feast of Sacrifice is an example of this practice (Bornstein, 1974).

6.2 FOOD AVOIDANCES

Food avoidances or taboos as part of the prevailing concept toward food may also influence distribution of food within the household. When dealing with food avoidances, for instance in relation to nutrition, it is useful to make a distinction between permanent and temporary food avoidances (e.g. de Garine, 1967).

6.2.1 Permanent food avoidances

We talk about a permanent food avoidance when a certain food may never be consumed. Permanent food avoidances are concerned with a whole population, a group or individuals. A classic example of a permanent food avoidance for a whole population is the avoidance of pork by Muslims. It often happens that restrictions on the consumption of certain foods are laid down for women. These restrictions on the consumption generally relate to the reproductive function of the woman and disappear when the woman has passed reproductive age.

6.2.2 Temporary food avoidances

Temporary food avoidances apply to individuals during certain periods within the life cycle: birth; pregnancy; lactation; childhood; various diseases. They concern the 'vulnerable' groups: pregnant women; breast-feeding women; the infant and the child during the periods of weaning and growth. Food regulations and avoidances during these periods are unfortunately often of the kind to deprive the individuals of nutritionally valuable foods such as meat, fish, eggs or vegetables. Most permanent avoidances have little effect on the nutrition of the individual, in contrast to the temporary food avoidances for individuals at certain critical periods of their life cycle. Food avoidances in nutrition has been somewhat overstressed compared with other aspects of food habits. It is very difficult to find out their origin as they have a long history. An introduction to the origin of flesh food avoidances in Europe, Africa and Asia, made by the geographer Simoons (1962), can be recommended.

28

6.3 INFANT FEEDING

Of all population groups affected by malnutrition, young children need most attention. Protein-energy malnutrition among young children and sometimes also vitamin A deficiency are still a severe problem in many developing countries. Practically always the underlying cause is a combination of dietary inadequacies, and chronic or repeated acute infections. Behind these two causes, there are various interrelated conditioning factors.
- A marginal food supply as a result of rural poverty.
- Both in town and country, income is not sufficient to purchase food for a nutritional adequate diet. Poor households have to spend at least 70% of their income on food that often hardly meets their energy requirements.
- Because of commercialization of the rural areas and rising prices, particularly in towns, many mothers are forced into money-earning activities, often in the informal sector. This means long working hours, low income and an increase in the burden of work for mothers at the expense of child care. In the poorer households, income is far too low for making adequate arrangements for child care during work.
- Food habits may sometimes aggravate the situation, e.g. unequal apportionment of food in the household. The weaning period, i.e. when the child is gradually or abruptly taken off the breast and given other foods, has become identified with the overwhelming problems of protein-energy malnutrition and other deficiency diseases (Cameron & Hofvander, 1976). The culturally prescribed weaning foods in traditional societies are usually soft carbohydrate foods, meat, vegetables and fruits playing no significant role, although these may be available and consumed by other family members. In improved weaning diets, nutrition education should have a major role but the actual practices must be fully understood before attempts are made to modify feeding practices, as well as the underlying economic and socio-cultural reasons for these (Bornstein & Kreysler, 1972).
- Hygienic conditions in many places are weak and there is a lack of safe drinking water. This is a point of major concern when introducing weaning foods.

- There is some evidence that advertising and marketing by the infant food industries have damaged infant feeding practices.

A common reason for infant malnutrition, especially in urbanizing areas, is the tendency to replace breast-feeding by artificial feeding soon after birth (Figure 5) (Raphael et al., 1979; UNICEF, 1981). Infants receiving sufficient breast milk run no risk of protein--energy malnutrition up to an age of about 6 months, provided that no complications set in and that breast milk represent an important part of the diet up to 2 years. Prolonged breast-feeding is still common practice among lower socio-economic classes in rural areas of developing countries.

Among these groups there is no satisfactory alternative to breast-feeding. Milk substitutes are either in short supply or too expensive, and poor hygiene makes artificial feeding, especially bottle feeding, extremely hazardous for the health of the baby. Ebrahim (1978) has calculated that the average cost of artificial feeding an infant in a developing country can vary from a quarter to a third of the official national minimum wage

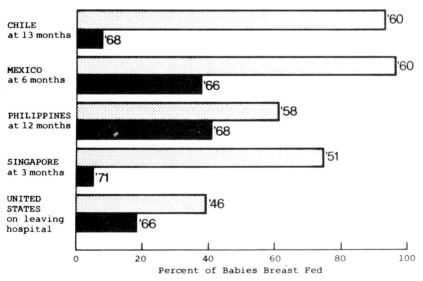

Figure 5. Decline in breast-feeding in some developing countries. From Ebrahim, 1978, Fig. 5.5.

Table 5. Cost of artificial feeding an infant 6 months old for a day in the United Kingdom and some developing countries. Data from Ebrahim, 1978, Table 6.3.

	Minimum wage ($ (US) per week)	Cost of feeding ($ (US))	Proportion of wage (%)
United Kingdom	39.20	1.30	3.3
Burma	5.01	0.81	16.2
Peru	5.60	1.30	23.2
Philippines	9.69	2.59	26.7
Indonesia	5.60	1.62	28.9
Tanzania	7.62	2.44	32.0
India	4.62	1.62	35.1
Nigeria	5.18	2.44	46.1
Afghanistan	2.80	1.62	57.9
Pakistan	5.18	3.23	62.4
Egypt	4.09	2.59	63.3

(Table 5). So adequate artificial feeding is beyond the reach of the poor mothers.

Turning away from breast-feeding is not only expensive for the poorer households but also for a country. Several attempts have been made to calculate the economic value of breast-feeding. Almroth & Greiner (1979) have estimated for the Ivory Coast that if every infant were breasted for two years, the savings in national costs could amount 16 to 28 million US dollars annually. If it declined to the level of the breast-feeding in Paris in 1955, the annual national cost would be between 33 and 55 million dollars. Though breast-feeding in Western countries is increasing, mainly for psychological reasons, after having shown a decline beginning in the 17th and 18th Centuries (Wood, 1955) the opposite trend is unfortunately spreading in the developing countries (Jelliffe, 1968; Thomson & Black, 1975). It must be realized that information on the causes of decline of breast-feeding are still scanty.

Breast-feeding habits may vary greatly within a country, as shown by three studies in Ethiopia (Knutsson & Mellbin, 1969). In one agricultural community without noteworthy signs of economic and social change, the duration of breast-feeding was long: 92% of the children were breast-fed for a year or more. The second community followed the same pattern, but where changes occurred in economic status the period of breast-feeding was shorter in those households. In the third community, infants were weaned in order to increase the number of children born to a women during her fertile years. In some societies, sexual intercourse is not permitted during lactation and the diminishing of polygamy has led to a decrease in the period of breast-feeding.

Several studies have shown the decline in breast-feeding in urban areas. In Chile, breast-feeding at one year of age fel in 20 years from 95% to 6% (Mönckeberg, 1965). In Yemen, a sample of women working at a factory stopped breast-feeding completely 8 months and many two months after a birth, whereas in rural areas 1½ to 2 years is common. Of working women, 85% used bottle-feeding, though this is still uncommon in villages (Bornstein, 1974).

Although the influence of advertising on behaviour patterns may be somewhat exaggerated in industrial countries (McKenzie, 1964), the consumer in developing countries is much more receptive to persuasion to use "modern" items and methods. The role of the infant food industries in developing countries has been much criticized in recent years. Numerous examples can be cited of aggressive advertising at the expense of breast-feeding. In order to establish a code of ethics on advertising and marketing of breast-milk substitutes and weaning foods, WHO and UNICEF organized a meeting in October 1979 on that topic with representatives of the food industry, science and countries. Two of the recommendations were as follows. Marketing of breast-milk substitutes and weaning foods should be designed not to discourage breast-feeding. No staff paid by companies producing or selling breast-milk substitutes should be allowed to work in the health-care system in order to avoid the risk of conflict of interest.

There is some evidence that an increase in domestic duties and paid work outside the home is an underlying factor in the decline in breast-feeding by poorer mothers (Popkin & Solon, 1976; Savané, 1980; Vis & Hennart, 1978). Advertisement for breast-milk substitutes have further aggravated the situation.

The position of children in non-Western society is rather different from that in Western societies. In Western societies,

the child does not belong to the adult world, hardly partici-
pates in nor shares duties in the activities of the adults. In
non-Western and rural societies, children form part of the world
of adults. At a very young age, they bear responsibility for the
daily basic needs of life, such as production and preparation of
food and taking care of younger brothers and sisters.
Children are expected to switch as soon as possible to adult
diets.

Numerous schemes for protein-enrichment of food have been
carried out in developing countries with varying success (Orr,
1972). These new food mixtures are based on local foods. Although costing much less compared with the imported infant foods,
they are still too expensive for poor households (Orr, 1977).
Food mixtures for relief of malnutrition can only reach poorer
infants as part of a government-subsidized nutrition programme.

7 Dynamics of food habits

7.1 CHANGES IN FOOD HABITS

The food habits and dietary pattern of a society are never static. They change with the socio-economic system of which they form part. A major aspect of the dynamics of food habits is the diffusion and acceptance of food crops and animals throughout the world. Trade, wars and migration have contributed in part to new foods. In the past 400 years, the transference of foods from one people to another has been extensive (Harlan, 1976; Niehoff, 1967).

From the Americas, maize, "Irish" potatoes, sweet potatoes, cassava, cocoa, tomatoes, Lima beans, groundnuts and turkeys went to Europe, Africa and Asia. Products like rice, tea, sugarcane and many fruits spreaded from South and South East Asia to other tropical and subtropical areas of the world. In many countries, these imported foods are so well established that people consider them indigenous. For Africa, Schnell (1957) estimated that 50% of the food crops originated from the Americas.

The new foods have had a considerable influence on the societies where they have been accepted. Cassava, with its high yield of energy has on many occasions saved populations from famine, despite its low protein content. In Indonesia and parts of East Africa, the cultivation of cassava was promoted as a hunger crop at the expense of rice and sorghum. The potato has played a similar role in Europe. According to Salaman (1949), it enabled the labourers to survive on the lowest possible wage when foods such as bread, meat and milk moved out of reach of the low economic classes. When maize was brought across the Atlantic, it became very well established in several countries around the Mediterranean, to some extent replacing wheat. Maize is a more drought-resistant crop and gives a higher yield.

Until quite recently, it was the food of the poorer sections of society in the Mediterranean (Chick, 1968).

In Mexico, Central America and northern parts of South America, traditional diets of the indigenous people are based on maize and beans. However one may observe a swing towards bread and rice; the same applies to parts of Brazil and in some of the tropical regions of Andean countries, where cassava is a staple food.

Another aspect of the dynamics of food behaviour is the acceptance of bread in areas of Africa and Asia not growing wheat. The history of the production of wheat and bread consumption is very old, but the acceptance of bread outside wheat-producing areas is mostly recent. For instance in Ghana, Bosman (cited by Kilby, 1965 and Youngs, 1973) wrote in 1704 that bread was available at the local market of Elmina. In South and East Asia where rice is the predominant preferred cereal, bread is increasingly accepted. In a sense, the two cereals do not compete with each other, since rice remains the centre of the diet and wheat products are supplementary foods suited to urban conditions (Aykroyd & Doughty, 1970). Several factors are involved in the acceptance of bread and other wheat products such as biscuits. These include urbanization and the need for time-saving foods, the presence of large groups and expatriates with bread-eating habits, a substitute for rice in periods of hunger (for instance Sri Lanka) and repatriation of soldiers who acquired a taste for bread while serving abroad.

In the industrial countries of Europe, North America and Oceania, the trend has been opposite: consumption of bread has declined.
A general increase in purchasing power and the greater diversity of foods other than wheat products has led step by step to the adoption of a diet containing large amounts of meat, a high proportion of fat, and increased amounts of vegetables and fruit.

7.2 INDUCING CHANGE

Food habits are changing constantly, for better or worse, by external influence or by modification from within the society

itself. Mead (1962) remarked: "The question we should be asking
is not how do we change food habits but how do food habits
change?" Indeed, it is only with a knowledge of existing trends
and interrelations of food habits and dietary patterns with other development trends, that one can hope to introduce those
changes that are nutritionally desirable and necessary.

Change of food habits is, generally speaking, induced by major agencies, each with its own objectives and methods:
- government institutions (e.g. Departments of Health, Education, Agriculture, Applied Nutrition Programmes) and voluntary
welfare organizations aiming to promote good food habits for better nutrition, generally through extension and nutrition education;
- commercial companies and agricultural marketing boards (both
private and state-owned) aiming to increase the demand for certain foodstuffs, with consequent need to change food habits
through promotion of these foodstuffs.
Often the interests of these two agencies do not coincide but
may conflict. For example, advertising may promote the use of
powdered milk for infants whereas nutrition education tries to
induce mothers not to abandon breast-feeding at too early a
stage. In industrial countries, consumption of sweets is highly
promoted, though nutrition education tries to reduce intake of
sweets and sugar in order to decrease the incidence of dental
caries. To avoid such situations, it is necessary to integrate
the aims and methods of the change agencies in a coordinated
food and nutrition policy of the central government, so that
they will not compete but rather complement each other. Unfortunately, such an approach is still wishful thinking in most countries, both industrial and developing.

Very often a change in food habits is induced by special nutrition programmes. The planning and evaluation of applied nutrition programmes is well described by Latham (1972). Before
starting to induce change, it is not only necessary to know the
food habits but also the trend of the food pattern. Generally,
the introduction of foods are likely to be successful if they
fit in with the existing trends such as the acceptance of processed infant foods, convenience foods, and bread or biscuits in

countries not traditionally growing wheat.

The converse is also true: so long as there is a high increasing demand for a food (e.g. sweets), it is unlikely that nutrition education will succeed in reducing consumption. Nutrition education can learn much from the commercial experience in changing food habits. Nutritionists should work with sociologists, socio-psychologists, communication specialists, and food marketers. To induce a change in food habits one can distinguish four main stages (Colby, 1964).

- Examining the roles of different foods. To change a food habit, one must know strength and importance of different foods to the individual and its role in the total life of the individual.
- "Product" testing the food or foods whose consumption is to be increased. Where a new food has to be introduced, one must use the same techniques for testing reactions to it as are used in research on new commercial products.
- Propaganda for these foods, presenting them in the most persuasive way. Whether one is trying to promote eggs in Guatemala or fish flour in Mexico and whether one is going to use mass media or personal contact in nutrition education, the overall theme must be agreed first.
- The testing of techniques for the mass media and for personal contact. This is a very complex field and readers who would like to have a concise introduction to this topic are advised to study Colby's paper.

Nutrition programmes are carried out by "change agents". The change agent, in our case the nutrition or health educator, is an employee with the task of introducing the chosen innovations to the target population. The activities of the change agents form a two-way process as it involves the action of the agent on the target populations and the reactions of population to the agent in accepting or rejecting a new idea, such as changes in feeding practices or a new food. Niehoff (1966) in his publication on social change summarizes six primary variables impinging on the change process. These variables will be listed below and briefly discussed within the context of changing food habits (Sections 7.3-4).

7.3 ACTION OF THE CHANGE AGENT

How does the change agent communicate? In most nutrition
programmes person-to-person communication has so far prevailed
and the potentials of mass communication have been underutilized
(Fuglesang, 1974; Manoff, 1974; Parlato, 1974). Too often staff
have been recruited (both international and national) with no
background and experience in education. It is not realistic to
expect positive results from inadequately trained educators. If
the nutritional message has not been carefully selected as specifically feasible and acceptable for the target group to which
it is aimed. Nutritionists sometimes try to turn the general
public into amateur nutritionists by supplying all kinds of
theoretical knowledge on food rather than specific practical
advice. Experience has shown that most success is achieved when
only one idea is taught at a time. Also, in a given region, the
messages broadcast by different agencies (health, agriculture,
education, community development) should complement and reinforce each other (Davey & McNaughton, 1969).

What kind of participation does the change agent obtain
from the target population? An often heard complaint from nutrition workers trying to influence a community to modify its feeding practices and consumption patterns is that the people are
conservative, backward and "resistant to change". The idea of
rural communities especially as fatalistic and conservative is
a die-hard image among scholars and development workers alike.
This theory has often been disproved and reflects more the attitudes and approaches of the agent than the behaviour of the local people. If people are unwilling to listen and follow advice,
they usually have good reason, although these may seem irrelevant and mistaken to a nutritionist. One reason may be that the
extension worker is identified with the ruling elite, which
makes communication very difficult (Bantje, 1976).

How does the agent utilize and adapt his innovation to the
existing cultural pattern? One cannot say that the food habits
of a community or a group of persons are wrong. Many food habits
are adapted to the prevailing ecological conditions. In regions
where the keeping of livestock is very difficult or traditional-

ly unknown, small animals such as rodents and various insects and snails are consumed. The practice of many peoples in the Near East not to drink fresh milk but to take sour or curdled milk or milk in the form of yoghurt substantially reduces the number of pathogenic organisms that would be taken in with uncooled fresh milk. In an island in the Caribbean, nutrition education aiming at an increased milk consumption for children was based on the habits of drinking coffee with a little milk at breakfast and had some success. Attempts to get children to drink a glass of fresh milk, as is common in North America, failed.

7.4 REACTION OF THE TARGET POPULATION OR RECIPIENT

Did the recipient or target population feel an initial need? Too often, nutrition projects are imposed on communities from above without asking the wishes and ideas of the people concerned or recognizing their own efforts and endeavours. There is much talk nowadays in development agencies about self-help programmes and participation of the local people. It is recognized that no real change can take place without the active participation of the community. However such aspirations are difficult to be achieved and the easier "do as you are told and you'll see the results" approach is often resorted to.

Does the recipient perceive any practical benefit from adopting a change? The nutrition extension worker wants to achieve better health for the community through food habits, but the villager often has no means of perceiving how the nutrition programme will really benefit him or her.

Are local leaders brought into the planning and implementation of the process? Local leaders and public administrators must be actively involved. Without the genuine interest of policy-makers and public administrators, nutrition programmes will have limited success. Those nutrition programmes that were most successful had all been well grounded in the administrative structure of the country and received good support from the target population concerned (e.g. McNaughton, 1975).

8 Food and nutrition policy

Besides biological variables, a great variety of socio-economic, cultural and environmental variables influence food intake and nutritional status of any group of people (Chapters 2-7). Food and nutrition is part of the whole social structure and environment, so that nutritionists cannot solve nutritional problems alone. The ultimate solution lies in the formulation and implementation of a food and nutrition policy. Food and nutrition should be considered as an integral part of national development, as emphasized by an FAO/WHO expert committee (1976). During recent years several countries have given more systematic attention to these approaches.

It is not within the scope of this field guide to deal exhaustively with the complexities of food and nutrition planning (e.g. Berg, 1981; Joy & Payne, 1975; Lynch, 1979). However it is useful to list some crucial elements of such a policy.
- Nature and extent of nutrition problem(s).
In other words, who is malnourished, in what ways, in what circumstances and why? For example, is it a protein-energy or a vitamin A deficiency, among preschool children or landless labourers, chronic or seasonal? Is it because of certain beliefs, lack of sufficient land or unemployment?
- Selection of the target group. Which categories of the society should be covered by the policy? One may think of the vulnerable groups, low income households, deprived rural areas or shanty-town dwellers.
- Identification of relevant measures. Any development plan will include programmes having important nutritional effects, and programmes designed specially for their nutritional objectives. Programmes having large nutritional effects are agrarian reform, irregation schemes, introduction of new crop varieties and improvement of food storage. Programmes designed specifically for their

nutritional objectives may likewise include a wide range of activities: food rationing, food subsidies, supplementary food and
feeding programmes, maternal and child health activities, applied
nutrition programmes and nutrition education.

Data are needed as a basis for formulation and implementation of a food and nutrition policy. This should involve not
only the various planners at the central and provincial levels
but also persons and institutions coming from or working with
the target population.

9 Some notes on field studies

When you have been decided whether information is needed as part of a general survey or to solve a specific problem and which groups are to be surveyed, the design of the survey can be made. Before planning any survey, you must collect any existing information on the target population. More information than is first thought is sometimes available. This may be in books, articles in professional journals and reports of governmental institutions. Little of this information will be available on the spot. You can trace much of it through abstracting journals such as Nutrition Abstracts and Reviews, and World Agricultural Economics & Rural Sociology Abstracts, and current bibliographies such as Agrindex. These printed secondary sources should be available in at least a central library in the country where you are working and are also available as computerized data bases in regional centres.

You may also obtain useful information from local workers in agriculture and nutrition. Information from these informants may, however, be biased. You should contact a specialist or someone familiar with social surveys, if such a person is available, for advice and guidance.

9.1 FOOD HABITS AND FOOD CONSUMPTION SURVEYS, AN OUTLINE OF STEPS INVOLVED

A survey on food habits and food consumption involves several steps (just as in any social survey).

(1) Defining the problem

A. What is the precise formulation of the question (problem) to be answered?

B. What facts struck you and made you ask the question?

C. What is the goal of the survey?

(2) Survey methods to be used

A. What facts or data do you have to collect in order to answer
   your question (problem)?

   Demographic   : date of birth
                     sex

   Socio-economic : education
                     occupation
                     income
                     religion
                     language

   Food habits   : kinds of food
                     amounts of foods
                     food avoidances
                     food preferences
                     knowledge of food
                     foods given to infants

B. How should you collect data?
   The choice of method depends on the source and kind of facts
   or data you have to collect.

   Source   Methods

   Documents : studies, reports,   content analysis
               files
               ready made
               statistics   reprocessing of data

   Informants: local leaders   interviews
               field workers

   Population: (a) Observation:
                                           non-participant observation;
                                           to observe specific social
                                           situations concerned with
                                           food, but not to take part
                                           in it

                                           participant observation;
                                           one is a temporary insider
                                           by taking part in the vari-
                                           ous activities

                                           (b) Interview:
                                           personal interview
                                           personal interview aided by
                                           a questionnaire
                                           group interview

(3) Sampling

A. Choice of time of year:
   agricultural season
   market cycle
   periods of fasting

B. Sampling of the area:
   country/town/shanty town
   cash crops/subsistence crops
   ecological zone (forest, savanna)

C. Sampling of population:
   random sampling: theoretically equal chance of being chosen,
   e.g. every tenth or fiftieth from a list of households or
   from a map
   stratified sampling: samples with common characteristics,
   e.g. small farmers, landless farmers, urban workers, educated
   mothers

(4)   Organizing the survey, which includes:

A. Careful instruction or training of interviewers
B. Informing the population of the survey

(5)   Actual collecting data in the field

A. Pilot or trial survey in order to test out the survey method
B. Actual collecting of data

(6)   Tabulation and presentation of findings

(7)   Reporting

9.2   SAMPLING OF THE POPULATION

   In selecting rural communities and their members for the
study of food habits the following points should be taken into
account: the choice of the time of the year, sampling of the
area and sampling of the population.
   Food behaviour depends heavily on the time of the year. It
will be different before and after harvest (agricultural season),
and during feasting or fasting (religious cycle). The market
cycle may influence food behaviour too.
   Sampling of the area depends on where one needs to survey,

for instance countryside growing cash crops or subsistence crops, an industrial or a market town. The following aspects should also be considered:
- The ecological zone in which the community is situated, such as savanna or forest zone (climate and vegetation), lowlands or high plateau (relief and terrain).
- The socio-economic status of the community, for instance subsistence or cash crops, proximity to urban areas, and links with the outside world.

After you have selected the community or communities and the time of the year to carry out the survey, you must consider the population as such. Usually surveys of every individual are not possible because of time and effort. You must take a sample of the population.

Sampling is quite a complicated matter, preferably planned in collaboration with a statistician as there is always a risk of introducing a bias in the sample. There are several methods of sampling (e.g. Réh, 1976).

One method is that of random selection when theoretically every household has an equal chance of being chosen. If you, for instance, want to sample a rural community, you can choose at random one in so many households, depending on the size of the sample. Perhaps you can first make a map of the village with all its houses, then pick out one household at random, taking for instance every fourth or every tenth household. For the purposes of a survey, household may be defined as the group of persons eating from one cooking pot.

During the actual survey, you must record households that you chose but that refuse to take part, and also record the reasons given for refusal by the householders. If you believe the reasons given are not true, you should record that too. Such information may later be useful in helping to decide whether the sample was in fact biased in spite of efforts to obtain a random sample.

9.3 METHODS OF COLLECTING DATA

There are several methods of collecting field data. If you are associated with a food and nutrition programme and need information on the sociological aspects of food and nutrition, the following two methods are appropriate
- observation of the target population and its environment;
- personal interviews aided by a questionnaire. Each method has its advantages and weaknesses so that a combination is much better. A survey based on a structured questionnaire should be complemented with observation of the community (Sieber, 1973).

Observational methods of data collection are techniques for gathering information by watching the behaviour of individuals without direct questioning. This method, much used in social-anthropological surveys, may give useful information on food habits of a community and its members. A disadvantage is that it is time-consuming. In order to observe food habits adequately, one needs to stay for a long time in the community whereas food and nutrition programmes usually need information quickly. Another disadvantage is that only small communities can be observed adequately and the collected data are often difficult to process statistically. Items of data that may be observed are listed in Appendix A. More material on the item that may be included are given in Grivetti (1981), Guthe et al. (1945), Jerome et al. (1980), Leroi-Gourhan (1973), Mauss (1971), Murdock et al. (1950), and Notes and queries on anthropology, 1954.

Observational methods should be combined with personal interviews where the interviewer asks questions and records the answers on a questionnaire. This method allows one to collect numeric data, and is comparatively quick. A questionnaire has several limitations, the most important ones being: not all data can be collected by means of a questionnaire and persons interviewed may, for various reasons, withhold information.

Construction of a questionnaire is a complex matter (example in Appendix B). Careful attention should be given to the wording of the questions, which should be placed in a logical order. In asking a question, you should never suggest an answer. The different questions may be pre-coded or open, depending on the nature of the survey. A questionnaire often consists of a combination of the two kinds of questions. In pre-coded questions, the different possible answers are already mentioned in the questionnaire and the interviewer need only tick off one of them (e.g. Appendix B, Questions 2.8 and 2.9). Pre-coded questions can only be set if you know what answer might be given. This will not always be possible and then one needs an open-ended question so that the respondent's answer can be recorded (e.g. Appendix B, Questions 3.1, 3.2 and 3.3).

There is a natural tendency to introduce all kinds of items. Every additional question increases your work in the field and makes people less willing to cooperate. It also increases the work of tabulation and analysis. So questionnaires should be limited in length and scope to the essential information required. Only a fraction of the items included in Appendix A could be included in a questionnaire.

The illustrative questionnaire cannot be used as such, but is intended for adaptation according to the objectives and needs of the survey. The list of items of data on food habits (Appendix A) is a good source of material in developing a questionnaire. The questionnaire begins with demographic and socio-economic aspects of the household (Sheet 1). Only a minimum number of questions have been included. If the survey requires more information in this field, consult Appendix A2.

The other sections of the questionnaire deal with supply and preparation of food, distribution of food, infant feeding, food avoidances, special foods.

The questionnaire concludes with a section on the frequency of food consumption. This allows information to be collected on the kinds of food consumed and gives a picture of the dietary pattern of the target population. It is advisable to collect this information from a selected number of the target population after completion of the previous sections of the questionnare.

The situation becomes more complicated when a questionnaire must be translated into the local language. Often it is very difficult to translate certain concepts into another language. For instance, the concept 'food' differs greatly in various cultures. Questions can only be formulated adequately by someone

48

familiar with the local situation and idiom. Keep a detailed diary or notebook during a survey in order to record observations made on food and nutrition, and information received from various informants and the population.

9.4 FIELD WORK

Before starting a survey, the questionnaire must be tested and modified if necessary. The quality of the data depends heavily on the skill and conduct of the interviewer during the survey, rather than on the respondents. So selection and training of suitable interviewers is crucial for the survey. Is the interviewer a person likely to be accepted by the population and told delicate information, such as consumption of low-status foods? For the interviewers to be aware of the dynamics of an interview, they must practise, first by interviewing each other and then by a pilot trial. Interviewing each other will teach them the aims and methods of the survey much better, how respondents should be approached, how embarrassment about poor diets can be minimized and the importance of privacy during an interview to gain confidence.

The conduct of the interviewer during the survey may be summarized as follows:
- He should be fully familiar with the purpose and significance of the survey.
- He should have a good rapport with the respondent.
- He should have a large measure of respect for other people, regardless of social background and position.
- He should begin the interview with polite greetings and friendly conversation, but be careful not to talk too much.
- He should not suggest any answer for the questions to the respondent and should double check doubtful answers.
- Striking observations should be recorded.
- The collected information should be confidential.
- He should thank the respondent before leaving.

The target population should be well informed on the purpose of the survey and know that you wish to visit their homes to ask them questions. Collaboration should therefore be assured in advance from local leaders or representatives.

9.5 ACTUAL FIELD WORK

A number of problems are commonly encountered in collecting data. Local people are often suspicious of strangers and may therefore be unwilling to communicate with the interviewer. Such attitudes may be caused by previous unpleasant experiences. If they do talk to you, they may try to protect themselves by giving deliberately wrong information, or they may answer the questions rapidly without thinking, in order to get rid of you. Another more positive aspect that may be equally a problem is that many respondents may be anxious to please you and give answers they think are expected instead of reporting on their actual food habits. On questions related to food, such as on prefered or prestige foods, respondents may be confused between what they would like to eat and what they actually eat. People are often not used to respond to a whole range of questions and frequently retreat from the situation by stating they do not know or do not remember.

Each completed questionnaire should be carefully checked by interviewer or supervisor on the day the information is collected, to detect any inconsistencies, errors or incompleteness. At this stage of the survey, you can still visit the respondent again to check statements and to make corrections. After the field-work is finished, it is too late to do so.

10 Measurement of food consumption

The concept of food consumption to be measured, varies with the objectives of the survey. A report prepared by FAO (1977) distinguishes the following objectives:
- study of levels and patterns of food consumption and expenditure;
- calculation or revision of weighing factors for estimation of cost of living index;
- study of nutritional adequacy of diets in relation to requirements;
- study of the health and nutritional status of the population;
- other general objectives.
It is essential to distinguish between food consumption surveys mainly used for national food planning and administration and surveys whose emphasis is primarily on the relation between nutrition and health.

Distinction is necessary because each objective demands a different type of information. For the planning of food supply, one needs to know the demand and price of food, and farm incomes, so data are required on the amounts of foods taken from different distribution channels by various categories of users at different times (Section 6.1, Figure 4). The results of the survey should be expressed in terms of amounts of foods purchased. For economic analysis, there is less interest in what users do with food after it has been bought. If the study serves to assess the nutritional adequacy of the diet in relation to requirements or to assess the exposure to environmental chemicals through food, interest is in amounts of foods eaten. To assess the nutritional adequacy of the diet in relation to nutritional status, results are commonly expressed in terms of amounts of nutrients.

For each objective, various types of surveys exist and the approaches are at different levels:

- national accounts of annual food availability per head of population; food balance sheets;
- family budget and household consumption surveys;
- individual food intake or dietary surveys.

10.1 FOOD BALANCE SHEETS

Food balance sheet is a national account of the annual production of food, changes in food stocks, imports and exports, and distribution of food over various uses within the country.

This account can be prepared on the basis of the calender year, the agricultural year or the crop year. The various uses are listed under the following headings: animal feed; seed; industrial uses; waste; and the net food availability for human consumption at the retail level. Per capita food availability is given for the total population actually partaking of the food supplies during the reference period, i.e. the population present within the geographical boundaries of the country at the mid-point of the reference period. In some countries, the per capita food availability refers to only the civilian population, that is armed forces are excluded. Per capita food availability is expressed in grams of food, energy and some of the nutrients.

Food balance sheets can give a nutritionist the following information:
- a rough indication of the adequacy of national food supply;
- food availability relative to other countries;
- trends in food supply if food balance sheets have been compiled over some years. However to interprete trends, one must be aware of interfering factors such as trends in different segments of the population (e.g. increase of the elderly).
Food balance sheets give no information at all about how the food supplies are distributed between different segments of the population. They do not indicate vulnerable groups in a population. Generally speaking this kind of information is not of much interest for those working in food and nutrition programmes.

10.2 BUDGETARY AND HOUSEHOLD FOOD CONSUMPTION SURVEYS

Main characteristics of budgetary (Section 10.2.1) and household surveys (Section 10.2.2) are as follows:
- The unit of observation and tabulation is a household or family group.
- Amounts of food purchased or (sometimes) eaten must be measured.
- Results are usually presented as averages for groups of households having a common set of characteristics. These types of
surveys do not usually consider food intake, since it may not
be feasible to measure consumption outside the home. They do
not indicate distribution of food within the family and so are
sometimes combined with individual dietary surveys.

10.2.1 Budgetary surveys of families

Emphasis is on income and expenditure. Little or no information is obtained on foods actually used in private homes. However, some countries try to exploit this method more fully,
adapting it to provide particulars of amounts of food consumed
as well as expenditure on food. A further expansion might classify foods, and include age, sex and occupation of people present at each meal. These extra data make nutritional evaluations
of the average food consumption of various categories of households possible. However this additional information might over-
burden a budgetary survey, which is usually already heavily
loaded with questions (FAO, 1977b).

10.2.2 Methods used to ascertain food consumption of the household

Currently there are four ways of collecting data on household food consumption (Burk & Pao, 1976).
- The weighed-record method aims to weigh or measure in household units the food supplies for the day or the meal in advance.
This is done during daily visits by field investigators. Foods
not eaten by the household members may not necessarily be sub-

stracted.

- The inventory method aims to record acquisitions and changes in food inventory of the household generally over a period of one week. At the beginning and end of this period an inventory is made of food in the house and all foods brought into the house during this period are recorded.

- In the list-recall method the interviewer uses a list of major food items in a structured questionnaire to help the respondent to recall the amount and price or purchase value of all foods used in the household in a specified period, usually seven days.

- The food-account method aims to record all food purchases and food brought into the household from other sources during seven-day period or longer. This measure assumes that there have been no significant changes in household food inventories.

In order to make a nutritional evaluation of the food consumption or food available for the different categories of households, results of the surveys are expressed as energy and nutrients. Instead of expressing intakes per household member, one can calculate adult equivalents (sometimes called consumption units). A drawback is that the basis for this system is based on energy requirement relative to that of an adult man. However for different age categories, the requirements of protein, some minerals and vitamins are not proportional to energy requirement (Table 6). Data from housechols surveys do not give information on the adequacy of the diet of different age categories. To obtain this information a more complicated type of survey is needed namely an individual dietary survey.

Table 6. *Example calculation Consumption Unit Requirement of a man (body weight 60 kg) and boy (22 kg) for energy, protein and iron. Protein requirement assumes a net protein utilization (NPU) of 60.*

	Energy		Protein		Iron	
	MJ/d	relative	g/d	relative	mg/d	relative
Adult man	11.8	1	57	1	10	1
Boy aged 7 years	8.4	0.75	40	0.8	8	0.8

10.3 INDIVIDUAL DIETARY SURVEY

Individual dietary surveys are needed when data on food intake need to be evaluated against other nutritional data such as
nutritional status.

Individual dietary survey methods may be grouped into four
main categories:
- Recall of past intakes
- Recording of present intake
- Short-cut methods
- Combinations

10.3.1 Recall of past intakes of individuals

Recall methods aim at eliciting actual past intakes as re-
membered at an interview or with a questionnaire for completion
by respondents. The principal procedures for recalling past intake of individuals are:
- 24-hour recall
- Dietary history

The 24-hour recall method aims to ascertain the food intake
of an individual during the immediately preceding 24 hours or
the preceding day by means of detailed questions. Food intake
is usually assessed in terms of household measures. This method
estimates the food actually eaten, as recalled from memory. The
interview is not very complicated and does not take much time
for either interviewer or respondent. If the procedure is re-
stricted to one interview per respondent, information is limited
to the food intake on one particular day, though day-to-day
variation can be high for most people. So 24-hour recall is
often used together with another method (Section 10.3.4).

The dietary history method uses several approaches to obtain
information from the individual about his average food intake
during a certain period of time. During interviews, the respondent is asked to provide information about his overall pattern
of eating and also to recall the actual foods eaten during the
preceding 24 hours. In addition, the respondent is asked to complete a checklist of foods usually consumed and a cross check of

all foods actually consumed in a 3-day period.

The dietary history method (Burke, 1947) is a technique for estimating usual dietary intake. The technique is based on the premission that everyone has a constant daily pattern in his food habit. The method was originally developed to measure diets over a period of time for research on human growth and development. The rationale was that clinical and laboratory signs and findings may result from long-term food habits. Current intake may not reflect usual intake and so may have less value in evaluating the nutritional status (Burke, 1947; Young, 1965). The interview technique to obtain a dietary history requires highly trained interviewers with nutritional background. The data may be collected by the question, "What do you usually have for breakfast?" sometimes coupled to, "What did you have for breakfast this morning?" The amounts are recorded in common household measures. The complete day is covered in this way. If an individual does not have a constant eating pattern, a dietary history cannot be compiled. The dietary history including a checklist of foods and a cross check of all foods actually consumed in a 3-day period may be appropriate in the assessment of nutritional status and is not a great burden for the participant. However the skilled interviewers are crucial.

Recall methods in general have the following disadvantages. Respondents must have a good memory and (for 24-hour recall) a well defined pattern of diet. The methods make heavy demands on the interviewer, who has to gain the confidence of the participant to make good estimates, avoid suggestion and judge the reliability of replies. To gain the confidence of any respondent, interviews should be arranged in the house of the participant rather than in a clinic, despite the extra time that takes.

Their advantages are as follows. There is satisfactory co-operation because the interviews are no great burden for the participants. Dietary history and cross-checking give a picture of food intake by a group over a period of past time. The 24-hour recall may give a more exact picture of the actual food intake of groups of individuals.

10.3.2   Recording of present food intake

The amounts of food eaten can be weighed or estimated in terms of household measures.

The weighing method assesses the cooked weights of the total portions of the meal served, the portion of each individual and left overs. Often the ingredients and amounts used in the preparation of dishes are also measured. According to the co-operation and capacity of the participants, this method requires varying degrees of supervision. Educated people can weigh items for themselves with a spring balance provided for this purpose. With less educated people, the actual weighing should be done by the field-workers. So the nutritionist has to spend several hours each day with the mother, which may cause some interference in the home. To what extend this alters food intake is difficult to determine. A compromise must be reached between close supervision with consequent interference with the home routine and very little (perhaps inadequate) supervision so as not to upset the home pattern.

A record in household measures is a list of all foods eaten by an individual during a specified period given in terms of household measures or compared in size to food models. For educated people, this method is less demanding than weighing; they can record food intake themselves. There is less precision in this process but closer cooperation (Marr, 1971). Supervision by a dietitian at the beginning and end of a period is necessary. At the end, a detailed interview is desirable to allow checking of amounts. Details overlooked or omitted reduce the accuracy with which measurements can be converted to mass. For less educated people, this method is not appropriate, because they cannot record and describe their portions. If a nutritionist has to do the work and to spend much time in the house with the mother, she could better weigh the foods.

Recording has the following disadvantages. It can usually be continued for relatively short periods (one week at most). It is a great task for the participants; not every individual is willing or able to weigh the diet or to record the daily intake in household measures. Recording may alter the usual pattern of intake.

Advantages are that it gives a fairly exact picture of the
actual food intake of a group. If weighing is continued long
enough, reliable information about food intake of an individual
might be obtained.

10.3.3 Short-cut methods

Recall and recording provide information about amount and
type of food eaten. Short-cut methods give information only
about the quality of the diet. With a short schedule for qualitative classifications of dietary patterns, this method permits
rating or grading of items into categories so that extremes can
be identified. The questionnaire consist of simple clearly defined questions which can be used by untrained staff or can be
included in questionnaires completed by respondents.

10.3.4 Combinations

All methods have specific advantages and disadvantages.
There is no best method for all purposes. Investigators should
carefully consider what the best method is for their purpose.
Very often a combination of two methods might give fuller information. For instance, a combination of a weighing record at
household level and 24-hour recall for individuals can give information on food purchases of different categories of households, on recipes and on the food intake of groups of individuals.
A combination of a dietary history and current recording gives
information of a food pattern in the past and a more exact picture of current food intake.

10.4 SAMPLE SIZE AND DURATION OF SURVEY

Results of several studies have shown that accurate estimation of total intake of energy and nutrients by the individual
cannot be obtained from a dietary record or dietary history. In
every group, individuals can be found whose energy intake is
twice as much on one day than another. Day-to-day variation in
energy and nutrient intake within an individual can be as large

Table 7. *Number of random 24-hour recalls for 95% probability that the sample average is within 20% of the true individual mean. Data from Balogh et al. (1971).*

	For half the population	For 90% of population
Energy	4	9
Carbohydrate	5	10
Starch	8	23
Sugar	11	23
Animal protein	11	27
Vegetable protein	7	13
Fat	8	23
Saturated fat	9	22
Oleic acid	10	30
Linoleic acid	23	44
Cholesterol	20	45

as variations between individuals. Some investigators have tried to estimate the number of days needed in order to obtain information about an individual's food intake with acceptable precision. Table 7 shows the results of a study on 71 Israeli male civil servants (Balogh et al., 1971). These employees were contracted on a random day once a month for a year in order to get information about what they had eaten on the preceeding day. The authors calculated from their data the number of recalls needed to estimate an individual's diet with 95% probability of being within 20% of the mean for the person. To fulfill this criterion for 90% of the population, the number of recalls needed ranged from 9 for total energy to 45 for cholesterol. Taking into account that this criterion is not very specific, the results of this study show also that accurate data on individual food intake can only be obtained in long surveys. Usually this is not feasible: too time consuming, too costly and very often it is not possible to motivate the participants for such an effort. There are no data or number of recalls necessary when food supply is limited.

However, the purpose of consumption studies in epidemiology is rather to identify or characterize groups of individuals by their intake. Adequate sample size and number of records per subject depends on the requires precision of the assessment of nutrient intake and thus on the within and between individual

variation in nutrient intake of the group. So a pilot study is
essential, if no data on these sources of variation are available
in the literature. To get a picture of variation of food intake
over the week or season, interviews should be distributed
equally over different days of the week or season.

For sampling, the help of a statistician should always be
sought and the sampling technique should be described carefully.

10.5 VALIDITY AND REPRODUCIBILITY

Investigators must try to assess how far a set of data measures what is intended. Validity of each method can only be
tested against another, for there is no absolute method of dietary assessment.

The weighing method (and more specified the duplicate portion
technique (Section 11.1.1)) has been taken as the nearest to
ideal, though the conditions imposed on the subjects may effect
their behaviour more than recall techniques. Relative validity
has been demonstrated for recording and recall methods (Young
et al., 1952). However it has been difficult to obtain valid
dietary histories from children and the elderly.

Reproducibility refers to variance of a measure or observation. The variance can be divided into two main components:
random response errors or technical errors, and true or biological variability. Response errors arise from:
- the construction of diaries and questionnaires;
- the motivation and ability of the investigator or field worker;
- the motivation and ability of the respondent;
- the interaction between investigators and respondent.
Biological variability consists of true between-person variability and true within-persons variability, the latter comprising of
variations which are independent of time and those which are
systematically related to the day of the week. To improve reproducibility, Beaton et al. (1979) stressed the importance of dis-
tinguishing between the various sources of variance true between-
person variation in 'usual' intake (that is inter-individual
variation), day-of-the-week-effect, and residual variation. Residual variation includes 'true' within-person variation (day-to-

day variation) intake and methodological random error, and it is commonly referred to as intra-individual variation. Reproducibility can be determined in a test-retest design using various statistical techniques. A synonym for reproducibility, commonly used by clinical chemists is precision. Another synonym is reliability. However the term reliable is also used in a wider sense, to refer to the quality of the study design.

11   Conversion of amounts of foods into nutrients

When the amounts of foods are known, they can be translated into amounts of nutrients. Energy and nutrients in the diet may be calculated with tables of food composition or can be chemically determined from duplicate portions, aliquots or by the equivalent composite technique.

11.1   CHEMICAL ANALYSIS OF FOOD

11.1.1   Analysis of duplicate portions

If the food eaten has been weighed, chemical analysis of a duplicate portion is accurate. However, this method is not absolute, since the duplicate analyzed is not necessarily identical to the portion eaten. Small items taken with or between meals might be overlooked. Furthermore the duplicate might be prepared differently, so that the person under survey perhaps eats less or different dishes from what he would normally (Pekkarinen, 1970). Analysis of duplicate portions is time-consuming, very expensive, and can be used only in a study with highly motivated subjects. Consequently, it is difficult to sample a population randomly for such a study. The accuracy of results is also influenced by errors due to chemical techniques. Although these errors are presumably relatively small compared to the sources of error in calculations from food tables, even the most accurate method is not absolute. In general, this approach is too expensive and therefore not appropriate to field surveys.

11.1.2   Analysis of aliquots

During survey, all food eaten is weighed and all beverages drunk are measured, and all aliquots (e.g. a tenth of all foods and beverages, except for water, consumed) are collected daily. Subsequently the bulked aliquots of the survey period are chemically analysed. This approach is probably less accurate than analysis of duplicate portions because with mixed dishes the aliquot samples are not necessarily identical to the foods eaten.

11.1.3 Equivalent composite technique

The equivalent composite technique consists of two parts. All foods and drinks consumed are weighed or measured, and recorded for the whole survey. Afterwards a sample of raw food equal to the mean daily intake by an individual during the survey period is taken for chemical analysis. Compared to aliquot sampling, additional sources of variation are, however, introduced. Firstly unprepared raw foods are chemically analysed instead of prepared foods. Secondly the foods analysed may differ qualitatively and quantitatively from the foods eaten. The approach brings organizational problems, since food samples can be composed only after dietary intake have been calculated. However this method also has advantages. The food samples are easy to collect and the approach is cheaper than the duplicate portions or aliquot samples (Pekkarinen, 1970).

11.2 USING FOOD COMPOSITION TABLES

Food composition tables list the nutrient and energy contents of foods. Many composition tables only give the nutrient content of raw foods but others include prepared dishes. Those who prepare food tables have difficulty in ensuring that the foods listed are representative. Difficulties arise even with unprepared agricultural products, but are much greater for manufactured foods and home-prepared dishes. This knowledge inevitable raises the question "Should we use these tables for determining the nutrient intake of individuals and groups of individuals?" Many comparative studies have been carried out and their conclusions are not unanimous.

According to Marr (1971), comparison can be made at different levels. For individuals absolute agreement between calculated and measured values cannot be achieved. However differences for most nutrients are almost constant. For groups of individuals, mean intakes showed small differences, but were sufficiently in agreement for most nutrients.

In general, calculations and measurements agree, if the food composition table used is compiled mainly from analytical data on local foods. So the food tables used must be matched to foods eaten, especially the staple foods and foods that supply specific nutrients that are under study. An example of calculations for nutrient intake are given in Appendix E.

12 Reporting data

When data have been collected, they must be tabulated and analysed. Tabulation is the summarization of results in the form of quantitative tables. Almost all the information collected by questionnaire can be presented quantitatively. Quantitative analysis of social situations is usually more convincing for policy-makers than a descriptive or qualitative approach.

The oldest method of tabulating data is by hand, straight from the questionnaire, by ticking off on a list each entry from the questionnaire. This is simple and useful, not requiring special equipment. If one needs to work with more than two variables it is quicker and easier, to use other methods such as punched cards. One must then discuss the questionnaire with a local specialist in data processing before the field work. Such a specialist will tell how the questions can be put onto punched cards for the local data-processing system. However to collect basic information on food habits of a few persons, hand methods may suffice.

12.1 PRESENTATION OF NUMERIC DATA ON FOOD HABITS

The findings of the survey may be presented in tables, graphs, maps, sketches and photographs. Most findings may be presented in tables but graphic presentation may make the data easier to understand.

A table has three main parts: the caption (including number, title and explanation), headings and the columns of the figures themselves. Every table should have a title, placed above the table and should define the content briefly and clearly. Explanatory detail may immediately follow the title or may be placed at the table foot. If the information is obtained from other studies, the source should be mentioned at the end of the caption.

Each table must be understandable independently of the text of the report (examples in Appendix D)

Many of the data on food habits can be presented either descriptively or quantitatively. The two forms of information should complement and not duplicate one another. The advantage of tables is that they reduce explanatory and descriptive statements, facilitate comparison and make it easier to remember data. For a good understanding of a food and nutrition situation descriptive and quantitative data should complement each other.

12.2 WORKING OUT TRENDS

If a base line is available, one can work out changes in food habits in an intervening period. To allow valid interpretation, one must compare earlier data with recent ones collected by the same method on the same target group, and compare them with data from a reference group (Figure 6).

A reference group should be as far as possible identical to the target group, but differ mainly in that it has not been covered by food and nutrition activities. Comparison of A_1 with A_2 tells us whether any changes in food habits have occurred over the intervening period. A number of questions arise from this: Is the change the result of a general improvement in economic situation of the district, region or nation? A result of favourable weather? Or a result of food and nutrition activities? It

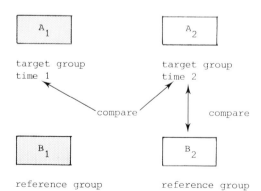

Figure 6. *Measuring change in community A.*

is necessary to look carefully into these questions.

To clarify the observed change, one must use a reference group.
Under ideal circumstances also from the reference group baseline data (B_1) should have been collected in order to detect change. Let us assume that the reference group B_2 differs much from A_2, but resembles both the base line situation of A_1 and B_1. The change in food habits may than result from food and nutrition activities in the district or region rather than from a general economic improvement. If there has been a general economic improvement, the reference group is likely to change in the same directions as A_2. In many cases, unfortunately, such base line data have not been collected. In order to get at least some idea on possible changes on food habits in an intervening period, one may compare A_2 with the reference group B_2. (Appendix C, table C20). However, working out trends and detecting intervening variables is a very complicated matter so that collaboration with a statistician is recommended.

12.3 PUTTING THE REPORT TOGETHER

There are of course several ways of preparing a report on field studies. For a report on a single field study on food habits and consumption along the lines we have discussed, the following successive elements are proposed:
- Abstract: all the bibliographic and indexing information needed by secondary services grouped around an informative summary. Policy-makers and administrators may need to read your summary, so do not make it too technical.
- List of contents.
- Introduction: general circumstances and reason for study, and reference to any earlier studies that have been published.
- Aims or objectives: reasons why the study was carried out.
- Survey methods: choice of methods for the survey, including time and place, and limitations of the survey.
- The community and its situation. The food habits and consumption of a community or part of a community, such as men, women or children, cannot be studied in isolation. The report should

briefly describe and discuss the social and physical environment, for instance the ecological zone, the socio-economic situation and the relation of the community to the outside world.
- Results of the survey: compiled around tables of data (Section 12.1) with discussion of their significance.
- Conclusions and (if appropriate) recommendations.
- Acknowledgments. As a courtesy and a token of gratitude, acknowledge assistance that contributed to the study.
- References. A reference should provide in clear and succinct form the elements needed to identify and obtain any written work cited.
- Appendix. Bulky material not forming part of the main line of argument may be placed at the end, for instance a glossary of foods and the questionnaire used.

Appendix A. Items of observational data on food habits

A1. SOCIAL GEOGRAPHY OF THE COMMUNITY

1. Type of community (village, suburb, quarter of a town, shanty town).
2. What are the means of existence of the community (subsistence farming,
cash cropping, fishing, industry, trade)?
3. Means of communication (main road, railway, waterway, airport).
4. Distance from nearest means of communication.
5. Vegetation zone.
6. Geographic zone (lowland, highland, mountain).

A2. SOCIAL STRUCTURE OF THE COMMUNITY

1. Social status of the survey group in the community (elite, middle class,
lower class, tenant, landless labourer, estate worker, caste, ethnic and
religious group).
2. Social services (schools; medical services including hospital, medical
doctor, public health nurse, or dispensary; social welfare programmes,
credit facilities, rural extension).
3. Food marketing services (a market, eating houses, shops selling food,
butcher, baker).
4. To what extent and how does the group use the services?
5. Are "traditional" medical practitioners and other traditional advisers
consulted on matters such as health?
6. Who owns the land, crops, livestock, fishing boats, workshops, industry,
houses and other resources?
7. Who decide on the political and economic affairs of the community inside
or outside the community?
8. Who are considered by the target population as their leaders (both male
and female)?
9. Are agricultural monetary resources in the community available such that
they cover the food needs (in the sense of energy) of all its members? If
not, does this apply for the whole community or only certain categories or
groups within it?

A3. FOOD PRODUCTION

1. What is the agricultural production system and land ownership (subsistence
farming, cash-crop farming, size of the farm, smallholdings, estates)?
2. What kind of agricultural implements and techniques are used (digging
stick, spade, pick, hoe, plough; irrigation, terrace cultivation, crop rota-
tion with fallow)?
3. Which agricultural and related tasks are carried out by men and which by
women?
4. What is the agricultural calendar?
5. What kind of crops are cultivated (staples, grain legumes, vegetables,
non-food crops)?

6. What kind of fruit-trees are grown?
7. What kind of livestock is kept?
8. What kind of fish is caught?
9. Method of fishing (netting, trapping, poisoning, angling)?
10. What kind of foods (animals and plants) are collected (food-gathering)?
11. What kind of animals are hunted or trapped for food and how?

A4. MEANS AND METHODS OF FOOD STORAGE

1. Kinds of food stored.
2. Where is the food stored (inside or outside the dwelling, in silos, pots or other means)?
3. Methods of preservation, i.e. smoking, pickling, fermenting, salting, drying (air, sun, mechanical).
4. Who owns the stored foods and who is in charge of the distribution?

A5. SUPPLY AND PREPARATION OF FOOD

1. What kinds of food are obtained from the individuals' own farm and from barter?
2. Who goes to buy food from the market, shops and other places?
3. What kind of foods and non-food items are purchased in the market?
4. Is food adulteration common practice and, if so, on which foods and how?
5. Who provides the market money for food?
6. Who fetches the fuel for cooking?
7. Who fetches the water for cooking?
8. Kind of water supply (piped water in the house, piped water outside the house, river, well and type, other; distance).
9. Is sufficient water available the whole year round?
10. What method is used to make a fire (matches, wood, friction, percussion, hammering)?
11. What kind of cooking stoves are owned and used (electric stove; electric stove with oven; gas stove; gas stove with oven; buta-gas stove; buta-gas stove with oven; kerosene stove; smokeless stove with oven; charcoal pot; tripod of stones or mud; separate oven made from mud; separate tin oven; hot box)?
12. What kind of kitchen utensils are available and what are they made of (pot, bowl, frying pan, cooking pan, dish, plate, cup, saucer, spoon, fork, knife, ladle, pestle and mortar for pounding grains or roots and tubers, small pestle and mortar of stone or wood, grinding stone: iron, clay, metal, stone, wood)?
13. What type of fuel is used for cooking (electricity, gas, butane gas, kerosene, coals, wood, charcoal, straw, dried cow-dung)?
14. Who does the cooking?
15. Who assists in preparation of food (daughters, wives, relatives, neighbours)?
16. Where is the food prepared (inside the dwelling, in the open, both inside and outside)?
17. What kind of foods and drinks are consumed?
18. How are the different kinds of food prepared (boiling; parboiling; stewing; steaming; baking; frying; grilling; roasting; smoking; salting; pickling; fermenting; rotting; drying in air, sun or machine; eaten raw)?
19. How are different drinks prepared (solution such as sugar or honey in water, suspension such as meal and water, extraction or treating with cold water, infusion with hot water such as tea, boiling, fermentation)?
20. Is earth eaten?

21. What kind of stimulants are used to increase vital and intellectual activities (coffee, tea, cocoa, kola, nuts, mate, quinine bark, betel, areca nut).
22. What kind of narcotics are used to produce lethargy or stupor and relief of pain (opium, coca leaves, qât leaves, Indian hemp)?
23. What kind of digestives are used?

A6. DISTRIBUTION OF FOOD AT HOUSEHOLD LEVEL

1. How many meals a day are served, at what time or after which kind of work?
2. What are the different eating groups during the time.
3. Who is responsible for distribution of food within the household and in each eating group?
4. Does each member of the household eat from his own plate?
5. Do the members of the household eat from a common plate or pot?
6. Is it the habit to wash hands before eating?
7. Is food eaten with the hands?
8. If not, what eating instruments are used (fork, spoon, knife, chopsticks)?

A7. FEEDING OF INFANTS (UP TO THREE YEARS OF AGE)

1. How long is breast-feeding continued?
2. Is breast-feeding given on demand of the child, according to a schedule, or according to maternal inclination?
3. Do women have sexual intercourse during lactation and, if sexual intercourse is avoided, why?
4. At what age is the first food other than breast milk given (weaning)?
5. What was the first food other than breast milk, and what is the method of feeding (cup, cup and spoon, feeding bottle, hand, chewing by mother)?
6. Is breast-feeding increasingly replaced by milk products such as: powdered milk, evaporated milk, sweetened condensed milk? If so, why?
7. Do present duties and responsibilities allow mothers to give sufficient time to breast-feeding and other forms of infant care?
8. Are promotional activities for infant foods going on in the community, and if so, which kind?
9. Why did the mother stop breast-feeding?
10. Was breast-feeding stopped at once or gradually?
11. How is breast-feeding stopped?
12. What kind of special foods for infants (weaning) are prepared or bought?
13. Who takes care of the child and especially feeding (the mother or guardian)?

A8. FOOD AVOIDANCES

1. What kind of foods and drinks may not be consumed by the following categories: infants during weaning; girls, boys, women during menstruation; women during pregnancy; women during lactation; all women; all men?
2. For what reasons are these foods and drinks avoided?
3. What kind of foods and drinks may not be consumed during illness by adults, by children?
4. What kind of foods may not be consumed during religious feasts, or other special occasions.

A9. SPECIAL FOODS AND DRINKS

1. What kinds of special food and drink are consumed by pregnant women?
2. What kinds of special food and drink are consumed by lactating women?

3. What kind of foods and drinks are prepared, purchased or given for: birth of a child; puberty rites of boys; puberty rites of girls; wedding; funeral; sowing or planting ceremonies; harvest ceremonies; other occasions or feast days?
4. What kind of foods and drinks are offered to (distinguished) guests?

A10. WHAT DO PEOPLE THINK ABOUT

1. What kind of foods and drinks do women consider the best and what kind do they consider less good for husbands, wives, pregnant women, lactating women, breastfed children (supplementary foods), infants during weaning, pre-school children, sick children, sick adults, old people?
2. What kind of plants, animals or part of animals are considered unfit for consumption and why?
3. Is there a system how people classify their own foods?

A11. FOOD HABITS DURING FAMINE

1. What kind of foods were consumed during the last period of food shortage?
2. What was the nature of the food shortage:
   a. seasonal, such as a pre-harvest shortage
   b. non-seasonal, but occurring from time-to-time such as a bad harvest
   c. non-seasonal, but very rare
   d. other
3. What kind of foods, if any, are consumed during famine?
4. Are there any particular foods only consumed during famine?
5. Are unusual substances such as bark or clay used as food during famine?
6. By whom is a household supported during famine?
7. Are the number of meals a day reduced during famine?

A12. FOODS PREFERENCES

1. What kinds of food and drink do men and women most like to eat?
2. For what reasons are these foods and drinks preferred?
3. What kinds of food and drink do men and women not like to eat?
4. For what reasons are these foods and drinks not liked?
5. What kinds of commodity both food and non-food would men and women like to buy if sufficient money were available?

Appendix B. Example of a questionnaire on food habits

B1. HOUSEHOLD MEMBERS

This sheet deals with the composition of a household and the questions should be asked to the head of the household. A household is defined as persons eating regularly from the same pot.

The questionnaire is divided in two subsections and the first one (1.1) will give information on the demographic and the second one (1.2) on the socio-economic background of the household and its members. These are possible variables which may influence the food habits. At the top fill in the name of the place, address of the household or a short indication of the situation of the house. In some countries each house has a number. After the section has been checked carefully, the signature of the supervisor. Do not forget to give the date of the interview.

B.1.1. Demography

Code number. Each member of the household will be given a code number to be used throughout the questionnaire.
Name of each member of the household.
Relationship to head of household. Place ach person on a separate line and list the persons in the followin~ order:
1. male head;
2. female head;
3. unmarried children from the oldest to the youngest (mention the relation to the head of the household, son or daughter);
4. other family members. Start first with married children, their spouses and children;
5. other members of the household such as employees or boarders.
Sex. Male or female.
Date of birth: age. If known, state date of birth and calculate age in completed years. Often age has to be estimated, which may be quite a complicated matter. Often national census reports give informations on how to estimate the age of persons who cannot give accurate information on their date of birth.
Marital status. Indicate if applicable, 1st, 2nd wife, married, unmarried, widow(er), divorced.

B.1.2. Socio-economic information

Code number, name. Repeat as on Sheet B1.1.
Ethnic group. If applicable, indicate which ethnic group or tribe each person belongs to.
Religion. The religion to which a person says he belongs.
School standard: final level at primary or secondary school, or other educational institution. If a person did not receive any formal education but can read and write, state as literate and the language in which he or she is literate.

Place: .... Address: .... Name of field-worker: .... Date: ....

Signature supervisor ....

B1 HOUSEHOLD MEMBERS

B1.1 Demography (information from head of household)

Code No	Name	Relationship to head of household	Sex	Date of birth	Age (years)	Marital status
1						
2						
3						
4						
5						
6						
7						
8						
9						
10						

<u>Main occupation</u>. This is when more than half the total working hours are devoted to one occupation. If no occupation, place a dash (-).

<u>Other occupation</u>. When less than half the total working time is devoted to another occupation. Sometimes the information received may be rather confusing, e.g. a person may state that he is a driver, while in actual fact, he is a farmer and driving is only a subsidiary occupation. Careful questioning may be needed to distinguish the main from other occupations.

<u>Employment status</u>. This may be stated as self-employed, government-employed, employed by a private firm or unemployed.

<u>Place of work</u>. This may be in the community itself, elsewhere at a stated place.

B1.2 Socio-economic information (information from each person)

Code No	Name	Ethnic group	Religion	School standard	Main occupation	Other occupation	Employment	Place of work
1								
2								
3								
4								
5								
6								
7								
8								
9								
10								

B2. SUPPLY AND PREPARATION OF FOOD

(Information from women responsible for food preparation).

Often these questions may be asked of the wife of the head of the household. If more than one women is responsible, for instance a second wife, a second sheet of the questionnaire should be used. Bear in mind that assisting in food preparation is not the same as being responsible for the preparation of food. Questions 2.1 to 2.7 may be answered by the family relationship of the person doing each task to the respondent. Name and code number are not required.

Name and code number of respondent	
2.1 Who fetches food from the farm?	
2.2 Who buys food from the market?	
2.3 Who receives food by barter?	
2.4 From whom is the barter received?	
2.5 Who provides the money to buy food?	
2.6 Who fetches the fuel for cooking?	
2.7 Who fetches the water for cooking?	

2.8 Who helps you in preparing the food?
 	
    - daughter(s)
    - co-wife (ves)
    - relative(s)
    - neighbour(s)
    - others (stated) ....
	□
	□
	□
	□
	□

2.9 Is food prepared?
 	
    - inside the dwelling
    - in the open
    - both inside and outside
	□
	□
	□

B3. DISTRIBUTION OF FOOD

(Information from person(s) responsible for food preparation)

    If more than one person is responsible for food distribution, a second
sheet should be used. Question 3.1 is concerned with the eating groups during
meal time (Section 6.1, Figure 4). It is necessary to know who is responsible
for the distribution in each eating group in order to understand the distribution system (Question 3.2 and 3.3). Of equal importance is to know the
order in which food is received (Question 3.4) by the household members and
whether the food is eaten from a common dish or each from his own plate
(Question 3.5).

Name and code number of the respondent	
3.1 With whom did the members of the household eat yesterday?	
3.2 Who is responsible for general distribution of food during meal time and in each eating group?	
3.3 Who is responsible for the distribution of food during meal time in each eating group?	

3.4 In which order is the food received by the members of the household? (indicate 1, 2, 3)
 	
    - husband
 	
    - wife
 	
    - son(s)
 	
    - daugther(s)
 	
    - others (stated) ....
	☐
	☐
	☐
	☐
	☐

3.5 Do members of the household eat from
        - the same dish or plate?
        - or own plate?
	☐
	☐

3.6 Is it usual to wash hands before eating?	

78

B4. INFANT FEEDING

(Information from mothers of children below 3 years of age, except in some societies where the guardian must be interviewed too)

In some societies, children may be placed in the care of a relative rather than with the mother. If so, the person responsible for the child should be identified and also interviewed if necessary. If there are more children below this age in the household a separate sheet should be completed for each, with the name and code number of the respondent, and the age and code number of the child.

	method of feeding[x]
Name and code number of the respondent	
Name, age and code number of the child of the respondent (below 3 years of age)	
4.1 Do you breast-feed your child now? (If not, go to Question 4.7)	

4.2 If so, when is breast-feeding given:
        - on demand of the child?
        or
        - according to schedule?
        or
        - according to your inclination?
	□
	
	□
	
	□

4.3 Do you give your child supplementary food as well as breast milk?	□
4.4 If so, at which age did the child receive food other than breast milk?	------ months
4.5 What was the first supplementary food given to the child?	

| 4.6 What kind of foods (including beverages) are given to the child in addition to breast milk and by what method of feeding?

        [x]Code

    cs: cup and spoon
     c: cup
     b: bottle (feeding bottle)
     h: hand
    ch: chewing by mother

(Go to Question 4.11 or 4.12) | food   method | method of feeding[x] |

4.7 If not, at which age of the child did you discontinue breast-feeding?	------ months

4.8 Did you stop breast-feeding
 	
    - at once?
    - gradually?
	☐
	☐

4.9 How did you stop breast-feeding?	
4.10 Why did you stop breast-feeding?	
4.11 What kind of food do you now give to your child?	
4.12 Which of the foods given to the child are prepared or bought specially for the child?	Home prepared infant foods
	Purchased infant foods
4.13 Which of the foods given to the child are just ordinary adult foods?	Adult foods given to infants

80

B5. FOOD AVOIDANCES OR TABOOS

(Information from head of the household and if male also from his wife)

Generally food avoidances observed by the head of the household and his wife are decisive for the food habits of the household. If you are interested in food avoidance of the old and young generations, other members of the household can be interviewed as well. Fill in the name and code number of the respondents and record not only foods that should not be eaten but also the reason why.

Name and code number of the respondents				
Which foods and drinks may not be consumed by the following categories and why?	Kinds of food and drink	Reason	Kinds of food and drink	Reason
- Infants during weaning				
- Girls				
- Boys				
- Women during monthly periods				
- Women during pregnancy				
- Women in general				
- Men in general				
- Sick persons				

B6. SPECIAL FOODS

(Information from head of the household and if male also from his wife)

Question 6.1 deals with special foods for pregnant and lactating women; Questions 6.2 and 6.3 with food and drinks for special occasions; Questions 6.4 and 6.5 with special kinds of food or unusual substances such as bark or edible earth, consumed during famine.

Name and code number of respondents		
6.1 Do women have special foods and drinks during	Kinds of food and drink	Kinds of food and drink
- pregnancy? - lactation?		

6.2 What kinds of food and drink are used for
 	
 - celebrating birth of a child?
 - puberty rites, boys?
 - puberty rites, girls?
 - weddings?
 - funerals?
 - sowing or planting ceremonies?
 - harvest ceremonies?
 - other (stated)
  ....
  ....
 		

6.3 What kinds of food and drink does one offer to distin- guished guests?		
6.4 What kind of foods are consumed during famine?		

B7. FREQUENCY OF FOOD CONSUMPTION

    Collect the information from a selected number of the target population.
The form is based on 24-hour recall and the list of foods printed on the form
should be extended if information is already available. For larger households,
two sheets will be necessary in order to interview more than four members.
Ask each member of the household, "What kinds of food and drink did you eat
yesterday?" For children, the mother or responsible person should be asked.
Unless otherwise required, collect the information on a "normal" day and not
on a feast day or other special occasion. For survey of food habits, respondents are asked only the kind and not the amount consumed. The collected data
gives the dietary pattern of the household and its members. Accurate quantitative information is difficult to collect by recall in rural areas of developing countries.
    If there is a pattern of three meals daily, the information should be ob-
tained separately for the morning meal (M), noon meal (N) and evening meal
(E). A three-meal pattern is not universal. Place a cross in the heading M,
N or E when that meal is the main one of the day. Snacks should also be recorded by including it in the nearest meal or adding a new column concerning
snacks to the questionnaire. List all the foods consumed in the left column,
ant tick them off under the column M, N and E. State also the origin of the
food as bartered (B), home-produced (H), gift (G) or purchased (P). Describe
the food consumed as completely as possible. For instance do not write down
only "cassava" or "meat", but also if it is dry or fresh, what types of meat
or fish, whether smoked, roasted or otherwise prepared. Dishes, such as stew
should be listed, together with the ingredients.

What kind of foods did you eat
yesterday? (24-hour recall)

All members of the household
(children included)

Day: . . . Month: . . . Year: . . .

M: morning   (breakfast)
N: noon   (lunch)
E: evening   (supper)

Origin code: B: Barter
             G: Gift
             H: Home-produced
             P: Purchased

Name and Code No of person interviewed																				
Kind of food	M	N	E	origin	M	N	E	origin	M	N	E	origin	M	N	E	origin
1 Cereals, roots, tubers (staple food)																
2 Grain legumes																
3 Veg./fruit																
Nuts																
4 Animal foods																
5 Fats/oils																
6 Beverages																
7 Other foods																

Appendix C. Presentation of data on food habits

Examples of how to present demographic and socio-economic data of a community are given in Tables C1-C21. There are of course several ways of presenting these data and the samples are only simple suggestions. Most of the tables give absolute figures. With large numbers it is useful to calculate the figures on a percentage basis.

The frequency of food consumption which will give the dietary pattern of a community or group is presented in Tables C9-C13. The dietary pattern is qualitatively expressed in terms of percentage and frequency of use of different foods. It gives the kind of food and not the quantity of food consumed. Thus for instance in Table C9 an entry of 29 against "cassava" means that some "cassava" was eaten in 29 out of 100 meals. The average number of meals per day is calculated by dividing the total number of meals eaten by the number of persons.

In Table C9 very detailed information is given. The same information can also be used to show the general dietary pattern, and to give information on dietary patterns of different groups such as adults - men and women - children and infants (Table C10).

In this section some examples are given on presenting data in the form of tables not requiring complicated techniques (Tables C14 to C 21). The tables presented here are obtained from a number of small scale field studies in which the author was involved.

Table C1. Absolute frequency of
sex in community with age.

Age (years)	Number	
	male	female
<1	6	6
1-3	19	18
4-6	18	17
7-9	16	15
10-12	14	13
13-15	11	12
16-19	12	13
20-39	41	42
40-49	13	13
50-59	9	8
60-69	5	6
>70	3	5
<1-70+	167	168

Table C2. Absolute frequency of
household size in community.

Number of persons in household	Number of households
1-2	5
3-4	10
5-6	16
7-8	10
9-10	5
11-12	5
>12	3
1-12+	54

Table C3. Age and sex of heads of households in community.

	Age (years)					
	20-29	30-39	40-49	50-59	60+	20-60+
Male	6	8	9	6	19	48
Female	-	1	2	1	1	5
Either sex	6	9	11	7	20	53

Table C4. Marital status of persons aged 16 years or more in community.

Age (years)	Male				Female			
	married	single	widower	total	married	single	widow	total
16-19	–	12	–	12	2	11	–	13
20-39	36	5	–	41	39	3	–	42
40-49	12	1	–	13	12	1	–	13
50-59	6	1	2	9	6	–	2	8
60>	5	1	2	8	5	–	6	11
16-60+	59	20	4	83	64	15	8	87

Table C5. Educational level of boys and men in community.

Age (years)	Illiterate or not attending school	Primary school only	Secondary school	Others	Total
4-6	9	9	–	–	18
7-9	2	14	–	–	16
10-12	1	9	4	–	14
13-15	1	4	6	–	11
16-19	4	3	5	–	12
20-39	10	28	3	–	41
40-49	10	–	2	1	13
50-59	7	1	1	–	9
60>	7	–	1	–	9
4-60+	51	68	22	1	142

Table C6. Educational level of girls and women in community.

Age (years)	Illiterate or not attending school	Primary school only	Secondary school	Others	Total
4-6	9	8	–	–	17
7-9	6	9	–	–	15
10-12	1	9	–	–	13
13-15	3	3	6	–	12
16-19	4	3	6	–	13
20-39	13	26	2	1	42
40-49	12	1	–	–	13
50-59	7	1	–	–	8
60>	10	1	–	–	11
4-60+	65	61	17	1	144

Table C7. Main and subsidiary occupation of men in the community, 16 years and older.

Main occupation	Number	Subsidiary occupation				
		farmer	trader	artisan	other	none
Farmer	50	+	4	5	2	39
Trader	8	5	+	–	2	1
Artisan	4	3	–	+	–	1
Other	2	–	–	–	+	2
Unemployed	19	1	–	–	–	18
Total	83	9	4	5	4	61

Table C8. Occupation of women in community, 16 years and older.

Occupation	Number
Farmer	60
Trader	2
Artisan	3
Other	1
Home-maker only	15
None	6
Total	87

Table C9. Dietary pattern in community, August over 7 days, about 80 people observed at each meal.

	Relative frequency (%) of foodstuff			
	any meal	breakfast	lunch	supper
Proportion of meals at which item was recorded (%)	87	90	80	90
Plantain	2	–	0.7	6
Cassava	29	3	8	76
Yam	2	1	1	3
Cocoyam	6	0.1	1	17
Maize	48	63	64	13
Bread	16	34	5	9
Doughnuts, Biscuits	2	4	0.9	0.3
Rice	7	22	4	4
Tomatoes	76	56	80	94
Onions	75	55	79	94
Peppers	76	58	81	94
Aubergine	19	10	16	33
Okra	8	5	12	9
Leaves	1	0.3	4	0.3
Fruit	0.3	0.1	–	0.3
Beef	12	5	10	21
Bushmeat	–	–	–	–
Pork	10	5	10	15
Mutton and goatmeat	11	2	8	24
Smoked meat	3	0.8	2	7
Chicken	0.7	0.3	0.3	1
Snails	0.4	–	–	1
Hen eggs	0.2	0.3	0.3	0.2
Fresh fried fish	8	9	12	5
Smoked fish	43	23	40	68
Salted fish	4	3	9	2
Tinned fish	0.2	0.1	0.7	–
Shrimps, Crabs	0.2	0.1	0.1	0.3
Milk (tinned)	13	27	3	9
Groundnuts	65	2	4	11
Beans	8	21	1	0
Palm nuts	11	4	7	21
Palm oil	4	0.8	10	0.7
Palm kernel oil	1	1	2	–
Groundnut oil	0	–	–	0.1
Coconut oil	10	19	8	3
Sugar	22	46	9	12
Sweets	0.6	0.5	–	–
Beverages including tea and coffee	12	25	2	8
Spirits	3	3	1	3
Salt	80	69	82	93

Table C10. Dietary pattern based on 100 meals of men (n=42) and women (n=38) in community, August.

	Relative frequency (%) in meals	
	men	women
Roots or tubers	43	37
Maize	49	59
Other cereals	22	27
Sugar	19	24
Vegetables or fruits	82	77
Beans including groundnuts	13	13
Meat	31	28
Fish	60	60
Other animal products	12	14
Palm nuts or oil	11	11
Other oils and fats	13	11

Table C11. Dietary pattern of the community, classed as home-produced and purchased (including gifts), 80 people interviewed.

	Relative frequency (%) in meals	Proportion of foodstuffs (%)	
		home-produced	purchased
Roots or tubers	40	74	26
Maize	45	3	97
Bread	16	–	100
Rice	7	–	100
Beans including groundnuts	13	1	99
Palm nuts or oil	11	–	100
Tomatoes	76	82	18
Onions	75	1	99
Peppers	76	93	7
Meat	30	4	96
Fish	60	–	100

Table C12. Dietary pattern based on 100 meals of socio-economic classes in community (n=80). The classes were defined as follows: high, big farmers and traders; middle, small farmers and artisans; low, landless labourers and squatters.

	Proportion of meals with foodstuff (%)		
	high class	middle class	lower class
Roots and tubers	32	40	48
Maize	38	44	52
Bread	30	15	4
Rice	25	6	1
Pulses including groundnuts	20	13	10
Vegetable oil	25	10	8
Tomatoes	76	74	70
Onions	78	75	72
Peppers	78	76	71
Meat	40	28	5
Fish	60	55	20

Table C13. Seasonal influence on dietary pattern in community (n=80).

	Proportion of meals with the item (%)		
	March	June	October
Roots and tubers	2	4	32
Maize	76	22	48
Millet	0	72	17
Rice	18	8	0
Pulses including groundnuts	18	8	0
Leafy vegetables	16	9	0
Other vegetables and fruits	2	1	0
Meat	51	13	0
Fish	21	22	81

Table C14. Members of urban and rural households responsible for supplying money used for purchases at market.

Place	Husband	Wife	Husband and wife	Children	Relatives
Town	9	7	3	1	–
Country	11	3	4	1	–

Table C15. *Members of urban and rural households responsible for buying food.*

Place	Husband	Wife	Husband and wife	Children	Relatives
Town	–	15	–	3	2
Country	–	14	–	3	2

Table C16. *Frequency of cooking in urban and rural households.*

Place	Once per day	Twice per day	Thrice per day
Town	6	8	6
Country	9	6	4

Table C17. *Persons doing cooking in urban and rural households.*

Place	Cooking alone	Cooking not alone					total
		other wife	daughter	female relative	husband	other	
Town	6	–	6	5	1	2	14
Country	6	2	8	2	1	–	11

Table C18. *Duration of breast-feeding in town and country.*

Place	Duration (months)					
	<3	3–5	6–8	9–11	12–17	>18
Town	–	–	2	1	7	3
Country	–	1	1	–	4	6

Table C19. Number of mothers giving supplementary foods to infants according to age and method of feeding in a rural community. (n=45).

	Age (months)						Method of feeding			
	3	3-5	6-8	9-11	12-24	>24	cup	spoon	feeding bottle	hand
Maize pap	1	16	20	–	3	–	4	29	1	6
Bread	–	–	2	–	–	–	–	2	–	–
Rice	–	–	2	–	1	–	–	–	–	–
Plantain (banana)	–	–	1	–	1	1	–	2	–	1
Yam	–	2	8	2	6	3	–	–	–	21
Cassava	–	–	1	–	2	1	–	–	–	4
Soup/stew	–	–	5	–	3	1	–	–	–	9
Fish	–	–	–	–	–	–	–	–	–	–
Meat	–	–	–	–	–	–	–	:	–	–
Milk (canned powdered)	–	6	3	–	–	–	2	3	4	–
Groundnuts	–	–	–	1	1	–	–	–	–	2
Hen eggs	–	–	1	–	1	–	–	–	–	2
Beans	–	–	3	–	–	–	–	1	–	2
Fruits	–	2	1	–	–	–	–	3	–	–
Beverages	–	–	3	–	–	–	–	3	–	–
Palm oil	–	1	4	1	2	–	x	x	x	x
Margarine	–	–	1	–	–	–	x	x	x	x

93

Table C20. Proportion of meals (%) with various foodstuffs in Community A (n=80) in 1975 and 1980, and Community B in 1980 (n=80).

Food	Community A		Community B
	1975	1980	1980
Roots and tubers	40	40	40
Maize	45	44	43
Bread	16	20	17
Rice	7	15	8
Beans including groundnuts	14	30	15
Palm nuts or oil	10	20	12
Leafy vegetables	20	40	22
Other vegetables and fruits	75	76	76
Meat	11	25	12
Fish	18	30	17

Appendix D. Questionnaire on food consumption of an individual

For those working in food and nutrition programmes and who do feel a need for data on food consumption it is recommended to take the following aspects into account:
- sample size;
- time in days needed to record dietary intake;
- season of the year;
- measurement of the amount eaten by various individuals of the population sampled.

The example given here is a schedule for a 24-hour weighing record for an individual and has been used in a survey on food intake by schoolchildren.

The model consists of 3 sheets:

D1 General information
D2 Record of food intake
D3 Record of food preparation

Sheet D3 and to some extent Sheet D1 are necessary to calculate with any precision the nutrients supplied by cooked dishes

D1. GENERAL INFORMATION

List names of members of the household with their age and sex. Indicate members eating particular meals outside the home as well as guests sharing any meal. The information on the questionnaire must be kept confidential, so remove names from the questionnaire as soon as possible. If more socio-economic information is needed, use the outline questions on food habits (Appendix B2 to B6), and the household members inventory sheet (Appendix B1.1 and B1.2).

```
                              Family name      :
                                   address     :
                              Respondent name   :
                                        age     :
                                     weight:
                              Interviewer       :
```

GENERAL INFORMATION

```
┌─────────────────────────────────────────────────────────────────────────┐
│  Code:                                                                    │
│  Date:                                                                    │
│                                                                           │
│  Persons in household by sex and age (specify children)                   │
│  Men                                       Boys                           │
│  Women                                     Girls                          │
│                                                                           │
│  Morning meal   time of day:                                              │
│                 absent      :                                             │
│                 visitors    :                                             │
│                                                                           │
│  Midday meal    time of day:                                              │
│                 absent      :                                             │
│                 visitors    :                                             │
│                                                                           │
│  Evening meal   time of day:                                              │
│                 absent      :                                             │
│                 visitors    :                                             │
└─────────────────────────────────────────────────────────────────────────┘
```

D2. RECORD OF A PERSON'S FOOD INTAKE IN A DAY

- In recording foods, describe them carefully, for instance whether milk is whole or skimmed and whether flour is coarse or fine.
- Weigh dishes and containers before food is put on them.
- Where possible, weigh the food "as purchased" and the edible part (a check on your data).
- It may be impossible to weigh meals taken outside the home. Foods and dishes should then be reported in number or sizes in domestic measures such as cups, cigarette tins, bottles and by cost. Investigators must weigh samples to find out the average weight per measure or find out how much of the food can be bought from that same source for the money spent.

Family code   :
Respondent code:
Date   :

Time	Kind of food	Weight of empty plate (g) m_1	Weight of empty plate and food (g) m_2	Weight of plate and leftovers (g) m_3	Net intake (g) (m_2-m_3)	Remarks

D3. FOOD PREPARATION BY HOUSEHOLD

For cooked dishes, weigh
- container or pan
- raw ingredients
- edible portion of each food
- cooked food in container or pan
- leftovers not eaten by any member of the household or guest during the day.

From this information, and the amount of the cooked food eaten by the respondent, the amount of each ingredient eaten by the respondent can be calculated. The number of persons sharing the dish are a partial check on the actual amount eaten by the respondent.

Family code   :
Respondent code:
Date   :

Name of prepared food: Weight of container or pan:

Name of ingredient	Weight before preparation (g) m_1	Weight of inedible parts (g) m_2	Net weight raw (g) m_1-m_2	Remarks

Total
Weight of pan and cooked food
Weight of pan and leftovers
Weight of pan
Weight of food eaten

A meat sauce is taken as an example of how to calculate food intake.

(Example meat sauce)			weight of pan: 500
Ingredients:	Weight (g) "as purchased"	Non edible part (g)	Net weight raw (g)
Tomatoes (sliced)	200	–	200
Onion (ground)	250	20	230
Minced fatty pork	50	–	50
Palm Oil	35	–	35
Water	200	–	200
Red Pepper	10	–	10
Total			1225
Weight of pan and cooked foods			1060
Weight of pan and leftovers			500
Weight of pan			500
Weight of food eaten			560

Assume the weight loss during cooking is due to the evaporation of water.

Persons sharing the dish: 1 adult male
                          2 adult females
                          2 children under 13 years of age.

Respondent: boy 8 years of age.
Amount eaten by the boy: 80 g.
This seems a reasonable portion as judged by total weight of the dish and number of persons sharing the dish.

Assumed that the components are uniformly divided in the sauce, the amount of each ingredient eaten by the boy is as follows:

Fraction of sauce eaten by boy is 80 g/560 g = 1/7
Intake of tomato = 200 g/7 = 28 g
Intake of onion = 230 g/7 = 33 g
etc.

Before calculating the nutrient value of prepared foods, check whether your food composition table gives data for cooked or raw foods.

Appendix E. Examples of calculation of nutrient intakes

E1. HOW TO USE THE WORKSHEET

Table E1 is a record for the boy 8 years old mentioned in Appendex D3. We use the same food preparation sheet of the sauce. During cooking, dry rice takes up twice its weight of water.

Table E2 converts food intake into intakes of major nutrients, calcium iron, vitamin A, vitamin B-1, B-2 and C. Conversion was based on Platt (1962) and
- "Tables of representative value of food commonly used in tropical countries" by B.S. Platt, MRC Special Report Series 302
- a local table based mainly on analysis for this survey, and other food composition tables.

Data might be calculated with a computer, a calculator, or without any special equipment. There should be agreement beforehand on the rounding-off of data. Work with more numbers behind the decimal point than the food composition table indicates is useless and meaningless.

If, for instance, 25 g of a food has been consumed and the food contained 19.8 g of fat per 100 g, it is obvious that the person obtained

$$\frac{19.8}{100} \times 25 = 4.95 \text{ of fat.}$$

It has become practice to round to the even integer preceding the 5. Thus in this case 5.0 g of fat. In the food record, the data also has been rounded off. Common practice is that amounts above the 10 grams are rounded to the next zero or five. Amounts of food below 10 grams are usually rounded to the nearest gram (without decimals). However this rounding should be considered carefully. Other rules may need to be made for nutrient-rich or energy-rich foods.

E2. EVALUATION OF THE RESULTS

It is beyond the scope of this guide to explain how to use dietary standards on nutrient requirements. A few remarks on the interpretation of dietary survey data will suffice.

First one cannot assess the boy's diet on the basis of one day (Table E1). Suppose we have 50 records for one day of schoolboys 8 years of age, then one can evaluate their food consumption as a group and compare data with nutrient requirements laid down by experts.

Table E3 lists means and standard deviations of intakes of energy and nutrients by preschool children in Matunguli and Mbiuni (Kenya) against requirements laid down by FAO/WHO (1974). Energy intake of the Mbiuni children is far below requirements. However without data on the nutritional status of those children (height and weight), we cannot conclude that Mbiuni children had too low an energy intake. If data on the nutritional status show that the quotient of weight to height or weight for age is low according to accepted standards, these low values for weights are most likely due to a diet or a deficiency of energy.

A frequency distribution of intakes would ascertain that distribution was normal.

Table E4 shows the contribution of various foods to the intake of nutrients by the same preschool children. This kind of table indicates which foods are most important sources of energy and nutrients. This information can be used for nutrition education programmes.

Table E1. Record of food intake by boy 8 years old.

DAILY FOOD RECORD				Family code : --	
				Respondent code: 020411	
				Date : 1978-08-05	

Time	Dish, food	Weight of empty plate (g)	Weight of plate and food (g)	Weight of plate and leavings (g)	Food intake (g)	Remarks
09:00	bread, white	150	200+	–	50	
	margarine	150	205+	–	5	
	peanut butter	150	215	–	10	
	tea	50	250+	–	200	
	sugar	50	260	–	10	
11:00	banana	–	150	30	120	
14:00	rice (highly milled)					
	cooked	150	525+	–	375	
	meat sauce	150	605	–	80	
17:00	soft drink	50	250	–	200	
	biscuit	–			10	
19:00	rice (highly milled)					
	cooked	150	525+		375	
	sardines in oil seasoning	150	550		25	

Table E2. Calculation of nutrient intakes.

Name ....
Number ....

Food and description	Weight (g)	Energy MJ	Protein total (g)	Protein animal (g)	Fat (g)	Carbohydrate (g)	Ca (mg)	Fe (mg)	Vitamins A (mg)	B1 (mg)	B2 (mg)	C (mg)
white bread	50	.	4	–	1	23	5	0.5	–	0.05	0.02	–
margarine	5	.	–	–	4	–	–	–	–	–	–	–
peanut butter	10	.	2.7	–	5	6	3	0.3	–	0.03	0.01	–
sugar	10	.	–	–	–	10	–	–	–	–	–	–
banana	120	.	1.2	–	–	35	8	0.6	0.04	0.06	0.06	12
rice (125+125)	250	.	17.5	–	–	200	8	2.5	–	0.15	0.08	–
tomatoes	30	.	0.3	–	–	1	1	0.1	0.02	0.02	0.01	8
onion	35	.	0.5	–	–	4	10	0.2	–	0.01	0.01	3
fat pork	7	.	1	1	5	–	1	–	–	0.06	0.01	–
palm oil	5	.	–	–	5	–	–	–	–	–	–	–
red pepper	1	.	–	–	–	–	–	–	–	–	–	–
soft drink	200	.	–	–	–	24	12	–	–	–	–	–
biscuit	10	.	0.7	–	1	8	3	0.2	–	–	–	–
sardines in oil	2.5	.	5	5	6	–	100	0.8	0.01	–	0.05	–
		6.6	31.9	6	22	311	151	5.2	0.37	0.38	0.25	23

Percentage of energy derived from protein, fat and carbohydrate

					Energy%
Protein	32 x 4	=	128	= (538 kJ)	8
Fat	22 x 9	=	198	= (832 kJ)	13
Carbohydrate	311 x 4	=	1244	= (5225 kJ)	79
			1570	= (6595 kJ)	

Table E3. Intake of energy and nutrients by preschool children in Matungulu and van Steenbergen, Nutrition and the Akamba Child, Amsterdam, Royal Tropical Insti

Area	Age (m)		MJ	Massic intake (KJ/kg)	KJoule	Protein (g)				Fat (g)
						vegetable	animal	total	kgBW	
Matungulu (n=11)		$\bar{x}$	3.46	393	3465	15.3	5.4	20.7	2.3	21
		$\underline{s}$	1.30		1300	9.7	2.5	10.2		5
		rec%		94					115^a	
	13-18									
Mbiuni (n=4)		$\bar{x}$	2.76	301	2761	11.8	5.7	17.5	1.9	12
		$\underline{s}$	0.85		851	7.0	5.0	4.5		9
		rec%		72					95^a	
Matungulu (n=7)		$\bar{x}$	4.60	435	4603	23.7	7.3	31.1	3.0	18
		$\underline{s}$	1.28		1279	7.8	4.2	5.6		8
		rec%		104					150^a	
	19-24									
Mbiuni (n=4)		$\bar{x}$	3.66	360	3660	19.3	4.5	23.8	2.3	16
		$\underline{s}$	0.88		883	7.1	4.0	8.2		3
		rec%		86					115^a	
Matungulu (n=14)		$\bar{x}$	4.61	414	4604	25.5	3.7	29.3	2.7	14
		$\underline{s}$	1.00		999	6.4	2.7	7.9		6
		rec%		99					135^a	
	25-36									
Mbiuni (n=5)		$\bar{x}$	3.92	377	3917	18.2	9.1	27.3	2.6	14
		$\underline{s}$	0.58		582	2.2	2.8	4.0		5
		rec%		90					130^a	

a. Based on safe level of protein intake having a relative quality score of 60.

...iuni, compared with recommendation (rec.) of FAO/WHO (1974). Adapted from W.M.
te. $\bar{x}$, mean; $\underline{s}$, standard deviation; rec., recommendation.

arbo-ydrate	Calcium (mg)	Iron (mg)	Retinol (mg)	Thiamin (mg)	Riboflavin (mg)	Niacin (mg)	Ascorbic acid (mg)	Body weight (g)
36	200	5.6	0.27	0.48	0.33	2.7	21	8860
64	84	3.3	0.12	0.29	0.15	1.3	8	
	44	86	108	104	52	36	105	
19	231	3.0	0.28	0.27	0.34	1.82	12	9210
60	166	1.0	0.34	0.07	0.20	0.50	14	
	51	43	112	59	54	24	60	
00	429	9.9	0.72	0.75	0.69	3.95	57	10550
60	152	3.5	0.6	0.19	0.20	0.93	38	
	95	141	288	163	110	52	285	
57	269	7.9	0.86	0.60	0.48	3.13	25	10175
41	205	3.0	0.61	0.21	0.28	127	16	
	60	113	344	130	76	41	125	
09	242	10.0	0.62	0.80	0.50	4.11	41	11070
44	140	3.7	0.92	0.24	0.26	1.13	34	
	54	143	268	154	69	48	205	
70	407	6.9	0.1	0.63	0.67	2.59	14	10400
25	111	0.9	0.06	0.08	0.16	0.36	13	
	90	99	40	121	93	30	70	

Table E4. Contribution (%) of various foods to total intake of energy and different nutrients by 76 infants. Adapted from W.M. van Steenbergen, Nutrition and the Akamba child, Amsterdam, Royal Tropical Institute, 1975.

	Energy	Prot.	Fat	Carb.	Ca	Iron	A	B1	B2	Nic.	C
Cereals											
Maize grain	2	2	1	2	.	3	.	3	1	4	.
Maize flour	51	50	18	61	7	66	.	62	21	42	
Wheat flour	2	2	.	2	.	1	.	1	.	2	.
Rice	1	1	.	2	.	.	.	.	.	1	.
Bread	1	1	.	1	.	1	.	1	.	1	.
Subtotal	57	56	19	68	7	71	.	67	22	50	.
Tubers											
Taro	1	1	.	1	1	2	.	2	1	2	2
Sweet potato	1	1	.	2	1	4	1	2	1	3	13
Irish potato	1	1	.	2	.	1	.	2	1	5	5
Green banana	1	.	.	2	.	2	8	2	1	2	6
Subtotal	4	3	.	7	2	9	9	8	4	12	26
Beans											
Pigeon pea	2	4	.	2	1	3	.	4	1	3	.
Dry beans	1	2	.	1	1	3	.	2	1	2	.
Fresh beans	.	.	.	.	.	.	.	1	1	1	.
Subtotal	3	6	.	3	2	6	.	7	3	6	.
Animal Food											
Cow milk	7	13	17	2	39	.	7	6	35	3	2
Goat milk	.	1	1	.	1	.	.	.	1	.	.
Sour milk	1	4	.	1	10	.	.	2	9	1	.
Breast milk	20	11	50	12	26	4	37	5	16	17	32
Egg	.	1	1	.	.	1	1	.	1	.	.
Meat	.	.	.	.	.	.	.	.	.	.	.
Subtotal	28	30	69	15	76	5	45	13	62	21	34
Vegetables											
Tomato	.	1	.	.	1	1	4	2	1	3	8
Onion	.	.	.	.	.	.	.	.	.	.	.
Cabbage	.	1	.	.	2	1	.	1	1	1	5
Sukuma week	.	1	.	.	2	3	5	1	3	1	12
Cowpea leaf	.	1	.	.	3	4	34	2	3	3	7
Amaranth	.	.	.	.	.	1	2	.	.	.	1
Subtotal	.	4	.	.	8	10	45	6	8	8	33
Fat											
Veg. cooking	2	.	10	.	.	.	.	.	.	.	.
Margarine	.	.	1	.	.	.	.	.	.	.	.
Ghee	.	.	.	.	.	.	.	.	.	.	.
Subtotal	2	.	11	.	.	.	.	.	.	.	.

	Energy	Prot.	Fat	Carb.	Ca	Iron	Vitamins				
							A	B1	B2	Nic.	C
Fruits											
Banana	.	.	.	1	.	.	.	1	.	1	1
Papaya	.	.	.	.	.	.	1	.	.	.	2
Lemon	.	.	.	.	.	.	.	.	.	.	1
Subtotal	.	.	.	1	.	.	1	1	.	1	4
Others											
Sugar	2	.	.	4	.	.	.	.	.	.	.
Sweet drinks	.	.	.	.	.	.	.	.	.	.	.
Grand total	96	99	99	98	95	101	100	102	99	98	97

References

Adepoju, A.; 1974. Migration and socio-economic links between urban migrants and their home communities in Nigeria. - Africa 43 (4): 383-396.

Almroth, S.; Greiner, T.; 1979. The economic value of breast-feeding, FAO, Rome.

Anderson, N.; 1964. The urban community: a world perspective. Hall, Rinehart & Winston, New York.

Annegers, J.F.; 1973. Ecology of dietary patterns and nutritional status in West Africa. - Ecology of Food and Nutrition 2 (2): 107-119.

Arriaga, E.E.; 1968. Components of city growth in selected Latin-American countries. - Milbank Memorial Fund Quarterly 46 (2): 237-252.

Aykroyd, W.R.; Doughty, J.D.; 1970. Wheat in human nutrition. FAO, Rome.

Balogh, M.; Kahn, H.A.; Medalie, J.H.; 1971. Random repeat 24-hour dietary recalls. - American Journal of Clinical Nutrition 24: 304-310.

Bantje, H.F.W.; 1976. Sociological aspects of nutrition education in Jamaica. Fitzgerald: 94-105.

Basta, S.S.; 1977. Nutrition and health in low income urban areas of the Third World. - Ecology of Food & Nutrition 6 (2): 113-124.

Beaton, G.H.; Milner, J.; Corey, P.; McGuire, V.; Cousins, M.; He, R.P.; Stewart, E.; Ramos, M.de; Hewitt, D.; Grambsch, P.V.; Kassim, N.; Little, J.A.; 1979. Sources of variance in 24-hour dietary recall data: implications for nutrition study design and interpretation. - American Journal of Clinical Nutrition 32: 2546-2559.

Berg, A.; 1973. The nutrition factor: Its role in the national development; portions with R.J. Muscat. The Brookings Institution, Washington, 290 pp.

Berg, A.; 1981. Malnourished people, a policy view. World Bank, Washington, D.C. - Poverty and Basic Needs Series, June 1981. 108 pp.

Blanhart, D.M.; 1971. Outline for a survey of the feeding and the nutritional status of children under three years of age and their mothers. - Journal of Tropical Pediatrics and Environmental Child Health 17 (4): 175-186.

Bornstein, A.; 1972. Some observations on Yemeni food habits. - FAO Nutrition Newsletter 10 (3): 1-9.

Bornstein,A.; Kreisler, J.; 1972. Social factors influencing the attendance in "Under Fives' Clinics". - Journal of Tropical Pediatrics & Environmental Child Health 18 (2): 150-158.

Bornstein, A.; 1974. Food and society in the Yemen Arabic Republic. FAO, Rome. - ESN: Misc/74/4.

Brisseau, J.; 1963. Les "Barrios" de Patare: faubourgs populaires d'une banlieue de Caracas. - Cahiers d'Outremer 16 (61): 5-42.

Burgess, A.; Dean, R.F.A.; 1962. Malnutrition and food habits, report of an international and interprofessional conference on food habits, Guernavaca, Mexico, 1960. Tavistock Publications, London.

Burk, M.C.; Pao, E.M.; 1976. Methodology for a large scale survey of household and individual diets. United States Department of Agriculture, Washington D.C. - Home Economics Research Report No. 40.

Burke, B.S.; 1947. The dietary history as a tool in research. - Journal American Dietetic Association 23: 1041-1046.

Cameron, M.; Hofvander, Y. (Protein-Calorie Advisory Group of the United Nations); 1976. Manual on feeding infants and young children. United Nations Organization, New York. 184 pp.

Chick, H.; 1968. Maize and maize diets. FAO, Rome.

Colby, C.W.; 1964. The role of the experimental psychologist. - Yudkin & McKenzie: 75-89.

7iéme Congrès International des Sciences Anthropologiques et Ethnologiques. 1970. Moscow. Le Congrès, Moscow, 1964.

Davey, P.L.H.; McNaughton, J.W.; 1969. Nutrition education in developing countries. - FAO Nutrition Newsletter 7 (3): 34-36.

de Esquef, L.; 1975. Food and Nutrition Education in the Primary School. - FAO Nutritional Studies No 25, FAO, Rome. 107 pp. References. 3rd printing.

de Garine, I.; 1962. Usages alimentaires à Khombole, Senegal. - Cahiers d'études Africaines 3 (10): 218-265.

de Garine, I.; 1967. Aspects socio-culturels des comportements alimentaires. Essai de classification des interdits alimentaires. - Maroc Medical 47 (508): 764-773.

de Garine, I.; 1969. Food Nutrition and urbanization. - FAO Nutrition News Letter 7 (1): 1-19.

de Garine, I.; 1971. Food is not just something to eat. - FAO Ceres, 4 (1): 46-51.

de Garine, I.; 1972. The socio-cultural aspects of nutrition. - Ecology of Food and Nutrition 1 (2): 143-163.

Dema, I.S.; den Hartog, A.P.; 1969. Urbanization and dietary change in Tropical Africa. - Food and Nutrition in Africa (7): 31-63.

den Hartog, A.P.; 1973a. Dietary habits of Northern migrant labourers in Accra, Ghana. - Voeding: Netherlands Journal of Nutrition 34 (6): 282-299.

den Hartog, A.P.; 1973b. Unequal distribution of food within the household; a somewhat neglected aspect of food behaviour. - FAO Nutrition Newsletter 10 (4): 8-17.

de Wijn, J.F.; 1978. Field guide for the assessment of nutritional health. Wageningen, International Course in Food Science and Nutrition, ICFSN Nutrition Paper (2): 42 pp. 2nd ed.

Documentation. 1982. Presentation of scientific and technical reports. Documentation. Présentation des rapports scientifiques et techniques. TC 46, 22 pp.

Dwyer, J.T.; Mayer, L.D.V.H.; Dowd, K.; Kandel, R.F.; Mayer, J.; 1974. New vegetarians. 65: 529-536.

Ebrahim, G.J.; 1978. Breast-feeding, the biological option. MacMillan, London.

Eckert, H.; 1978. Environnement intra-urbain des grandes villes africaines, pourquoi? - Revue Tiers-Monde, (Jan./Mars): 149-159.

Eckholm, E.P.; 1976. The other energy crisis: firewood. - Ecologist 6 (3): 80-86.

Everett, M.W.; Waddell, J.O.; Heath, D.B.; 1976. Cross cultural approaches to the study of alcohol. Mouton, The Hague.

FAO (Food and Agriculture Organization); 1970. Indicative World Plan for Agricultural Development: a synthesis and analysis of factors relevant to world regional and national agricultural development. FAO, Rome.

FAO; 1974a. Women, population and rural development, Africa, FAO, Rome.

FAO; 1974b. Equipment related to the domestic functions of food preparation, handling and storage. FAO, Rome. Various pagings.

FAO/WHO; 1974. Handbook on human nutritional requirements. - Rome, FAO Nutritional Studies No 28, Geneva, WHO Monograph Series (61).

FAO/WHO Expert Committee on Nutrition; 1976. Food and nutrition strategies in national development. FAO, Rome. - Ninth Report of the joint FAO/WHO Expert Committee on Nutrition, 64 pp.

FAO/Unicef/WHO Expert Committee; 1976. Methodology of Nutritional Surveillance. Geneva, WHO. - Technical Report Series No 593, 66 pp.
FAO; 1977a. The Fourth World Food Survey. FAO, Rome. - Food & Nutrition Series No 10, 128 pp.
FAO, Economic Commission for Europe Study Group on Food and Agriculture Statistics in Europe; 1977b. Report of the tenth session (3-7 Jan. 1977).
FAO; 1979. Women in food poduction, food handling and nutrition. FAO, Rome. - Food & Nutrition Paper No 8.
FAO; 1981. Wood energy. Special edition 1 and 2, - Unasylva 3 (131;133): 44; 52 pp.
Fitzgerald, T.K.; 1976. Nutrition and anthropology in action. Van Gorcum, Assen/Amsterdam, 155 pp.
Frankle, R.T.; Heussenstamm, F.K.; 1974. Food zealotry and youth: new dilemmas for professionals. - American Journal of Public Health 64 (1): 11-18.
Freedman, R.L.; 1973. Nutrition problems and adaptation of migrants in a new cultural environment. - International Migration 1 (1/2): 15-31.
Fuglesang, A.; 1974. Mass communication applied to nutrition education of rural populations: an outline of strategy. - PAG Bulletin 4 (1): 7-12.
Geertz, C.; 1963. Agricultural involution; the process of ecological change in Indonesia. Berkeley, University of California Press.
Gift, H.H.; Washborn, M.B.; Harrsion, G.G.; 1972. Nutrition, behaviour and change. Englewood Cliffs, New Jersey, Prentice Hall. 392 pp.
Grindal, B.I.; 1973. Islamic affiliations and urban adoptation: the Sisala migrant in Accra, Ghana. - Africa 43 (4): 333-346.
Grivetti, L.E.; 1981. Cultural nutrition: Anthropological and geographical themes. - Annual Review of Nutrition, Palo Alto 1: 47-68.
Gugler, J.; Gilbert, A.; 1981. Cities poverty and development. Urbanisation in the third world. Oxford University Press, Oxford.
Guthe, C.E.; Mead, M.; 1945. Manual for the study of food habits, Report of the Committee on Food Habits, National Academy of Sciences, Washington. - Bulletin of the National Research Council 3.
Gutkind, M.; 1974. Urban anthropology: perspectives of Third World urbanization and urbanism. Van Gorcum, Assen.
Hansen, H.H.; 1970. Fresh water, pearls and oils. - 7e Congrès International des Sciences Anthropologiques et des Ethnologiques 8: 180-183.
Harlan, J.R.; 1976. The plants and animals that nourish man. - Scientific American 235 (3): 89-97.
Harris, D.R.; 1969. Agricultural systems, ecosystems and the origin of agriculture. - Ucko & Dimbleby.
Hill, P.; 1978. Food farming and migration from Fante villages. - Africa 48 (3): 220-230.
Huizer, G.; 1973. Peasant rebellion in Latin America. Penguin, Harmondsworth, Middlesex.
Ingham, J.M.; 1970. On Mexican folk medicine. - American Anthropologist 72: 76-87.
Jelliffe, D.B.; 1966. The assessment of the nutritional status of the community. World Health Organization. - Monograph Series (53). Geneva, WHO. 271 pp.
Jelliffe, D.B.; 1968. Infant nutrition in the sub-tropics and tropics. WHO. - Monograph Series (19). Geneva. 335 pp.
Jerome, N.W.; Kandel, R.F.; Pelto, G.H.; 1980. Nutritional anthropology. Redgrave, New York. 422 pp.
Jocano, Landa F.; 1975. Slum as a way of life: a study of coping behaviour in an urban environment. University of Philippines Press, Quezon City.
Jones, S.M.; 1963. A study of Swazi nutrition. Institute of Social Research, University of Natal, Durban.

Joy, J.L.; Payne, P.R.; 1975. Nutrition and national development planning. - Food & Nutrition (FAO) 1 (4): 2-17.

Kilby, P.; 1965. Patterns of bread consumption in Nigeria. - Food Research Institute Studies 5 (1): 3-18.

Knutsson, K.E.; Mellbin, T.; 1969. Breastfeeding habit and cultural context. - Journal of Tropical Pediatrics 15 (2): 40-49.

Kouwenhoven, T.; 1970. Olfactory and gustatory problems: an introduction to the technological, nutritional and physiological aspects of the organoleptic assessments of food characteristics. - World Review of Nutrition and Dietetics 12: 319-376.

Kraut, H.; Cremer, H.D.; 1969. Investigations into health and nutrition in East Africa. IFO, München. - Africa Studies (42).

Latham, M.C.; 1972. Planning and evaluation of applied nutrition programmes. FAO, Rome.

Leach, E.; 1970. Lévi-Strauss, Fontana, London.

Leroi-Gourhan, A.; 1973. Milieu et techniques: les techniques d'acquisition, p. 66-128. Les techniques de consommation, pp. 142-198. Editions Albin Michel, Paris.

Lechtig, A.; 1976. The one day recall dietary survey: a review of its usefulness to estimate protein and calorie intake. - Archivos Latino Americanos 26: 243-271.

Lewin, K.; 1943. Forces behind food habits and methods of change, from: Guthe, C. and Mead, M. The problem of changing food habits, Report of the Committee on Food Habits. - Bulletin of the National Research Council No 108, Washington, National Academy of Sciences.

Lipton, M.; 1977. Why poor people stay poor: a study of urban bias in world development. Temple Smith, London.

Lloyd, P.; 1979. Slums of hope? Shanty towns of the Third World. Manchester University Press, Manchester.

Lowenberg, M.; Todhunter, B.C.; Wilson, E.D.; Feeney, M.C.; Savage, J.R.; 1968. Food and man. John Wiley and Sons, New York. 341 pp.

Lynch, L.; 1979. Nutrition planning methodologies: a comparative review of types and applications. - Food & Nutrition Bulletin 1 (3): 1-14.

Maltha, D.J.; 1976. Technical literature search and the written report. (2nd edition, about 1979). Pitman, London.

Mangin, W.; 1967. Squatter settlements. - Scientific American 217 (14): 21-29.

Malinowsky, B.; 1944. A scientific theory of culture and other essays. University of Carolina, Chappel Hill.

Manoff, R.K.; 1974. The effective use of mass media in nutrition education. - PAG Bulletin 4 (1): 12-17.

Marr, J.W.; 1971. Individual dietary surveys: purposes and methods. - World Review of Nutrition and Dietetics (Karger, Basel) 13: 106-164.

Mauss, M.; 1971. Manual d'ethnographie. Petite Bibliothèque Payot, Paris. p. 52-67 (Réédition de 1947).

McGee, T.G.; 1975. The urbanization process in the Third World, Bell, London.

McKenzie, J.C.; 1964. Food trends: the dynamics of accomplished change. - Yudkin & McKenzie.

McNaughton, J.; 1975. Applied nutrition programmes: the past as a guide for the future. - Food & Nutrition (FAO) 1 (3): 17-23.

Mead, M.; 1962. Culture change in relation to nutrition - Burgess & Lane. 50-62.

Mintz Ahmed, M.J.; van Veen, A.G.; 1968. Sociological approach to a dietary survey and food habit study in an Andean Community. - Tropical Geographical Medicine 20: 88-100.

Molony, C.; 1975. Systematic valence coding of Mexican "Hot" - "Cold" food. Ecology of Food & Nutrition 4: 67-74.

Mönckeberg, F.; 1966. Programmes for combating malnutrition in the pre-school child in Chile. - National Academy of Sciences; National Research Council, 168-177.

Murdock, G.P.; Ford, C.S.; Hudson, A.E.; Kenedy, R.; Simmons, L.W.; Whiting, J.W.M.; 1950. Outline of cultural materials. pp 18-27, New Haven Human Relations Area Files, Inc. 3rd edition.

Muséum National d'Histoire Naturelle, Laboratoire d'Ethnobotanique; 1967. Aide mémoire pour établir une fiche de travail sur le terrain concernant les plantes d'intérêt alimentaire. Paris. (Mimeographed).

National Academy of Sciences: National Research Council; 1966. Pre-school child malnutrition: primary deterrent to human progress. NAS/NRC, Washington.

Nelson, J.; Mandle, P.E.; 1978. Peri-urban malnutrition, a neglected problem. - Assignment Children (43): 25-46.

Niehoff, A.H.; 1966. A casebook of social change. Aldine Publishing Company, Chicago.

Niehoff, A.H.; 1967. Food habits and the introduction of new foods. - Journal of the Washington Academy of Sciences 57: 30-37.

Notes and queries on anthropology 1954 revised and rewritten by a committee of the Anthropological Institute of Great Britain and Ireland. Routledge & Kegan Paul, London. 240-257.

Obayemi, A.M.U.; 1976. Alcohol usage in an African society.- Everett et al., 199-208.

Olabisis Olusanya; 1977. Manual on food consumption surveys in developing countries. Ibadan University Press, Ibadan, Nigeria.

Oomen, H.P.A.C.; 1971. Ecology of human nutrition in nutrition. - Ecology of Food & Nutrition 1 (1): 3-18.

Orr, J.B.; 1936. Food, health and income. MacMillan, London.

Orr, E.; 1972. The use of protein-rich foods for the relief of malnutrition in developing countries: an analysis of experience. Tropical Products Institute, London.

Orr, E.; 1977. The contribution of new food mixtures to the relief of mal-nutrition, a second lack. Food & Nutrition (FAO) 3 (2): 1-28.

Painter, N.C.; 1972. The importance of dietary fibre, with special reference to diverticular disease in the colon. - Nutrition 26 (2): 95-109.

Parlato, R.; 1974. Advertising and mass communications: a model for rural nutrition information programs. - PAG Bulletin 4 (1): 17-18.

Pekkarinen, M.; 1970. Methodology in the collection of food consumption data. - World Review Nutrition Dietetics 12: 145-171.

Philips, B.S.; 1971. Social research, strategy and tactics. The McMillan Company, New York. 398 pp.

Pimentel, D.; Pimentel, M.; 1979. Food, energy and society. Arnold, London. 165 pp.

Poleman, T.T.; Perera, L.M.; Fernando, W.S.M.; de Mel, B.V.; 1973. The effect of income on food habits in Sri Lanka. - Nutrition Newsletter 11 (3): 9-29.

Popkin, B.M.; Solon, F.S.; 1976. Income, time, the working mother and child. - Environmental Child Health 22 (4): 156-166.

Pyke, M.; 1968. Nutrition surveys of eight regions in the Philippines: a dietary phase. - Philippine Journal of Nutrition 22. Cited in FAO ESH Fact Sheet Series p. 1.

Pyke, M.; 1968. Food and Society. John Murray, London. 178.

Quiogue, E.; 1969. Nutrition surveys of eight regions in the Philippines: a dietary phase. - Philippine Journal of Nutrition 22. Cited in FAO/ESH Fact Sheet Series p. 1.

Raphael, D. (ed); 1979. Breast feeding and food policy in a hungry world. Academic Press, New York. 332 pp.

Read, M.; 1966. Culture, health and disease. Tavistock Publications, London. 142 pp.

Reh, E.; 1976. Manual on household food consumption surveys. FAO, Rome. - Nutritional Studies (18): 96 pp.

Richards, A.I.; 1939. Land, labour and diet in Northern Rhodesia. Oxford University Press, London.

Ritchie, J.A.S.; 1979. Learning better nutrition. - FAO Nutritional Studies 20. FAO, Rome. 264 pp.

Royal Anthropological Institute of Great Britain & Ireland; 1954. Notes and queries on anthropology, 6th edition. Routledge and Kegan Paul, London. 240-257.

Sakr, A.H.; 1971. Dietary regulations and food habits of Muslims. - Journal of the American Dietetic Association 58: 123-126.

Salaman, R.N.; 1949. The history and social influence of the potato. Cambridge University Press, London.

Santos, M.; 1967. L'Alimentation des populations urbaines de pays sous-développés. - Revue Tiersmonde 8 (31): 605-629.

Savané, M.A.; 1980. Yes to breast feeding, but how? - Assignment Children No 49/50: 81-87.

Schnell, R.; 1957. Plantes alimentaires et vie agricole de l'Afrique noire. Larose, Editeur, Paris.

Sieber, S.D.; 1973. The integration of field work and survey methods. - American Journal of Sociology 78: 1335-1359.

Simoons, F.J.; 1962. Eat not this flesh: food avoidances in the Old World. Madison University Press, Wisconsin.

Sinclair, H.M.; Howat, G.R. (ed); 1980. World nutrition and nutrition education. Oxford University Press, Oxford. UNESCO, Paris. 226 pp.

Southall, A.W.; Gutkind, P.C.W.; 1957. Townsmen in the making. East African Institute, Kampala.

Thomson, A.M.; Black, A.E.; 1975. Nutritional aspects of human lactation. - Bulletin of the World Health Organization 52.

Trémolières, J.; 1973. Nutrition: physiologie, comportement alimentaires. Dunod, Paris. 618 pp.

Ucko, P.J.; Dimbleby, G.M.; 1969. The domestication and exploitation of plants and animals. Duckworth, London.

UNICEF; 1977. Local initiatives and modes of participation in Asian cities. Unicef, Paris. - Assignment Children No 40.

UNICEF; 1978. Malnutrition and the urban poor. - Assignment Children No 43. 127 pp.

UNICEF; 1981. Breast feeding and health. Paris. - Assignment Children No 55/56. 220 pp.

UNICEF; 1982. Social planning with the urban poor. Paris. - Assignment Children No 57/58. 219 pp.

van der Haar, F.; Kromhout, D.; 1978. Food intake, nutritional anthropometry and blood chemical parameters in 3 selected dutch schoolchildren populations. Thesis, Agricultural University, Wageningen.

van Steenbergen, W.M.; 1975. Nutrition and the Akamba child. Report of the Royal Tropical Institute, Amsterdam. Netherlands and Medical Research Centre, Nairobi, Kenya.

Vis, H.L.; Hennart, Ph.; 1978. Decline in breast-feeding: about some of its causes. - Acta Paediatric Belgica 31: 195-206.

Wilson, C.S.; 1979. Food, custume and nurture; an annotated bibliography on socio-cultural and biocultural aspects of nutrition. - Journal of Nutrition Education. Suppl. No 1, 11 (4): 211-263.

Wood, A.I.; 1955. The history of artificial feeding of infants. - Journal of the American Dietetic Association 31 (5): 474-482.

Young, C.H.M.; Hagan, G.C.; Tucker, R.E.; Foster, W.D.; 1952. A comparison of
    dietary survey methods. 1. Dietary history versus 7-day record. 2. Dietary
    history versus 7-day record, versus 24-hour recall. - Journal of the
    American Dietetic Association 28: 124-128; 218-221.
Young, C.H.M.; 1965. Comparison of results of dietary surveys made by dif-
    ferent methods. Proc. 4th Int. Congr. Diet., Stockholm. 119-126.
Youngs, A.J.; 1973. Wheat flour and bread consumption in West Africa: a
    review with special reference to Ghana. - Tropical Science 14 (3): 235-
    244.
Yudkin, J.; McKenzie, J.; 1964. Changing food habits. McGibbon & Kee, London.
    144 pp.